OXFORD MEDICAL PUBLICATIONS

Gastrointestinal Problems in General Practice

D1742851

Gastrointestinal Problems in General Practice

Oxford General Practice Series • 26

Edited by

ROGER JONES

Professor of Primary Health Care,
University of Newcastle upon Tyne

OXFORD NEW YORK TOKYO
OXFORD UNIVERSITY PRESS
1993

Oxford University Press, Walton Street, Oxford OX2 6DP

Oxford New York Toronto
Delhi Bombay Calcutta Madras Karachi
Kuala Lumpur Singapore Hong Kong Tokyo
Nairobi Dar es Salaam Cape Town
Melbourne Auckland Madrid

and associated companies in
Berlin Ibadan

Oxford is a trade mark of Oxford University Press

Published in the United States
by Oxford University Press Inc., New York

A catalogue record for this book is available from the British Library

Library of Congress Cataloging in Publication Data
Gastrointestinal problems in general practice/edited by Roger Jones.
p. cm.—(Oxford medical publications) (Oxford general
practice series: 26)
Includes index.
1. Gastrointestinal system—Diseases. 2. Family medicine.
I. Jones, Roger II. Series. III. Series: Oxford general
practice series: no. 26.
[DNLM: 1. Gastrointestinal Diseases. 2. Family Practice. W1
OX55 no. 26 1993/WI 100 G26365 1993]
RC801.G39   1993   616.3'3—dc20   93–20496
ISBN 0–19–262227–7

Typeset by Cambrian Typesetters, Frimley, Surrey
Printed in Great Britain on acid-free paper
by Biddles Ltd, Guildford and King's Lynn

Preface

It has been a pleasure to collaborate with friends and colleagues in general practice and hospital medicine in the production of this book. Most of the general practitioner authors are members of the Primary Care Society for Gastroenterology, which was founded in 1985 to promote good clinical care of gastrointestinal problems in general practice by supporting education and research. Many of the specialists who have contributed to the book have also been involved in the educational and research activities of the Society.

We have set out to provide an account of the gastrointestinal problems facing general practitioners in their everyday work, rather than to produce a condensed version of a large textbook. As well as dealing with common symptoms and particular patient groups, the book explores a number of topics, such as choice and availability of investigations, access to hospital-based services, the ways in which patients and doctors make decisions about gastrointestinal symptoms, the role of the primary care team in management, and the relationship between general practice and the hospital. Many of these issues are controversial and arguments surrounding them will continue as the National Health Service emerges from its present turmoil. Suggestions for further reading, including references to studies mentioned in the text, follow each chapter. Whilst our central aim is to provide guidance towards safe, effective, efficient, and sympathetic treatment of gastrointestinal disorders, we have also tried to stimulate debate and innovation, and to encourage a thoughtful approach to management.

Newcastle upon Tyne   R. J.
March 1993

Contents

Contributors

Jeremy Barnes FRCGP General Practitioner, 16 Cheltenham Road, Gloucester

Michael Bramble MD, FRCP Consultant Physician, Middlesbrough General Hospital, Middlesbrough, Cleveland

Duncan Colin-Jones MD, FRCP Consultant Physician, Queen Alexandra Hospital, Cosham, Portsmouth

Brendan Devlin MA, MD, MCh, FRCS, FACS Consultant Surgeon, North Tees General Hospital, Stockton on Tees, Cleveland

Michael Farthing MD, FRCP Professor of Gastroenterology, St Bartholomew's Hospital, London

Ian Forgacs MD, MRCP Consultant Physician, Department of Gastroenterology, King's College Hospital, London

John Galloway MRCGP, MRCP General Practitioner, Darkwood, St Augustine's Way, South Wootton, King's Lynn, Norfolk

Pali Hungin FRCGP General Practitioner, The Health Centre, Sunningdale Drive, Eaglescliffe, Stockton-on-Tees, Cleveland

Sanjeebit Jachuck FRCGP, MRCP General Practitioner, 377 Stamfordham Road, Newcastle upon Tyne

Oliver James FRCP Professor of Geriatric Medicine, University of Newcastle upon Tyne, Newcastle upon Tyne

Roger Jones DM, FRCGP, MRCP Professor of Primary Health Care, The Medical School, Framlington Place, University of Newcastle upon Tyne, Newcastle upon Tyne

Wendy Makin MRCP, FFR, RCSI, FRCR Consultant Physician, St Oswald's Hospice, Regent Avenue, Gosforth, Newcastle upon Tyne

David Murfin FRCGP General Practitioner, Brynteg Surgery, Ammanford, Dyfed

Christopher Rolles FRCP Consultant Paediatrician, Paediatric Medical Unit, Southampton General Hospital, Tremona Road, Southampton

Toni Rolles MRCGP General Practitioner, Bassett Wood House, Bassett Wood Drive, Southampton

Greg Rubin MRCGP General Practitioner, Health Centre, Trenchard Avenue, Thornaby, Stockton on Tees, Cleveland

Richard Stevens MRCGP General Practitioner, East Oxford Health Centre, Cowley Road, Oxford

Robert Walt MD MRCP Senior Lecturer and Honorary Consultant Physician, Queen Elizabeth Hospital, Birmingham

1 Gastrointestinal problems in the community and in general practice

Roger Jones and David Murfin

Gastrointestinal problems are frequently encountered by individuals, general practitioners, and hospital doctors. Diary studies have shown that problems related to the gastrointestinal tract are among the most common symptoms recorded by subjects; they represent about 8 per cent of all consultations in general practice, and account for a substantial number of hospital out-patient referrals and admissions. In the UK, annual death rates from colorectal cancer (16 000), peptic ulcer (4500), and gastric and oesophageal cancer (12 000) are high, and outnumber those from other diseases, such as carcinoma of the breast and cervix.

It is important to measure and understand the extent and pattern of gastrointestinal symptoms in the community and in general practice for a number of reasons. For example, if service provision of medical staff and facilities is to be responsive and sensitive to health needs, morbidity patterns in the general population and in primary and secondary care need to be measured carefully. More sophisticated data-collection techniques, for instance involving georeferencing, can enable local and district variations in morbidity, mortality, and health need to be identified and service planning to be undertaken accordingly. In relation to prevention and health promotion, an understanding of the experience of common symptoms by individuals, before they become patients, is crucial, and the factors associated with health-seeking behaviour are also of central importance in this respect. Many serious diseases of the gastrointestinal tract, in particular colorectal cancer, can be detected early, if not prevented. An understanding, for example, of patients' health beliefs about bowel habit and rectal bleeding is therefore vital in designing appropriate educational and screening programmes. Finally, as general practitioners become increasingly responsible for budgetary management, accurate measurement of the illness experience of their registered populations needs to be undertaken.

The natural history of many common conditions is still based on observations made in the hospital setting. Prospective studies of common disorders in the population and in general practice therefore offer an important approach to describing the clinical realities of primary care. Properly assembled cohorts of patients can be used for planned, prospective longitudinal follow-up, with clear end-points permitting accurate observations of the natural history of common disorders.

An awareness of the extent of symptoms in the community is also an important component of a patient-centred approach to medical care. The more we know and understand about our patients' morbidity experiences, their reactions to them, and the agendas they bring to our consulting rooms, the better we will be able to negotiate and plan appropriate management.

Finally, the study of clinical behaviour in general practice and at the interface between general practice and hospitals is also of prime importance. An appreciation, for example, of the variations in the behaviour of general practitioners in terms of resource utilization (prescribing, referral, and use of investigations) is fundamental when health-care planning on a larger scale is undertaken. One situation when this could be of particular importance might be the experimental merging of District Heath Authorities (DHAs) and Family Health Service Authorities (FHSAs), permitting unitary budgetary and clinical planning, and avoiding some of the difficulties associated with having two prescribing budgets and a tug-of-war between hospital and community care.

UPPER GASTROINTESTINAL PROBLEMS

Symptoms in the community

Upper gastrointestinal symptoms are extremely common in the general population; they account for 3–4 per cent of all consultations in general practice and for about 30 per cent of all patients seen in gastroenterology out-patient clinics. The principal symptoms are dyspepsia, upper abdominal and epigastric pain, heartburn and reflux symptoms, and nausea and vomiting. Although the frequency of these symptoms amongst individuals has been recognized for centuries, with descriptions of upper gastrointestinal disorders entering into the literature of most cultures, the first accurate estimate of the prevalence of upper gastrointestinal problems undertaken since the National Health Service was established was published in 1959 and carried out in London at a number of factories. In this study historical radiological criteria for the diagnosis of peptic ulcer were used to establish that about 30 per cent of the adult population surveyed had experienced significant dyspeptic symptoms in the study period of 12 months. In 1963 another important study, undertaken on a near-static population of men living in the north-east of Scotland, was published. Using a variety of sources of information to determine the prevalence of dyspepsia and peptic ulcer disease, similar figures to those published earlier were reported. The number of patients developing new dyspepsia was found to be roughly equal to those becoming symptom-free.

More recently, a number of studies of dyspepsia in general practice, whose principal aim was to determine the prevalence of organic lesions responsible for dyspeptic symptoms, rather than the prevalence of dyspepsia itself reported similar, if somewhat lower, figures to those obtained in the previous surveys.

The most recent large-scale estimates of the prevalence of upper gastrointestinal symptoms come from a series of studies carried out by a group working in primary care in Southampton. In a large multi-centre study involving five university departments of general practice (Southampton, Birmingham, Nottingham, Aberdeen, and Glasgow), the six-month period prevalence of dyspeptic symptoms was found to be 38 per cent, with remarkably similar figures in most of the centres studied, with the exception of Glasgow, in which the prevalence figure was 51 per cent. A number of features of dyspepsia in the general population were observed in this survey. In both men and women, the frequency of symptoms fell with age, whilst consultation rates with general practitioners rose. Social class was not itself associated with the prevalence of dyspeptic symptoms but was associated with the diagnosis of peptic ulcer disease, which was more common in lower socio-economic groups. There was considerable overlap between dyspeptic symptoms affecting the upper abdomen and reflux symptoms either simultaneously or at different times. In detailed interview studies with dyspeptic patients, it was clear that dyspepsia was part of a symptom-complex, with more than half the patients reporting reflux symptoms and postural dyspepsia, nausea, and abdominal distension, as well as upper abdominal pain. Other studies have confirmed further overlap between symptoms of dyspepsia and those of irritable bowel syndrome.

Classification of dyspepsia

Despite this frequent concurrence of symptoms, the recommendations of an international working party on the classification of dyspepsia are helpful in making initial decisions about diagnosis and investigation. This group has suggested that dyspepsia may be classified as follows:

(1) ulcer-like dyspepsia;
(2) reflux-like dyspepsia;
(3) dysmotility-like dyspepsia;
(4) idiopathic dyspepsia.

Ulcer-like dyspepsia is typically epigastric, with some of the clinical features seen in gastric and duodenal ulceration. Reflux-like dyspepsia refers to symptoms which are principally retrosternal, accompanied by regurgitation of acid and with significant postural elements. Dysmotility-like dyspepsia is associated with more vague abdominal symptoms, abdominal bloating, and also with lower bowel dysfunction. Unlike the first two, response to acid suppression is likely to be poor. Idiopathic dyspepsia describes digestive symptoms which do not fit well into any of these categories and may be due to other conditions, such as disorders of the biliary tract.

As well as the problems of symptom complexes and symptom overlap, diagnosis is made more difficult by poor correlation between the clinical history and subsequent findings on investigation. The predictive value of many of these symptoms is poor; reflux symptoms possess the greatest specificity and positive predictive value for a final diagnosis of gastro-oesophageal reflux disease (GORD), but the predictive values for ulcer disease of many 'typical' dyspeptic symptoms is often disappointing.

Clinical conditions causing dyspepsia

The clinical correlates of these symptoms are peptic ulcer disease, GORD, non-ulcer dyspepsia, and gastric and oesophageal cancer. The most common of these seen in general practice is non-ulcer dyspepsia; self-limiting dyspeptic complaints are common, frequently resolve on symptomatic treatment, and require no further investigation, whilst persistent and severe symptoms, which are discussed in other chapters of this book, require fuller evaluation.

The lifetime prevalence of peptic ulcer disease for adult males in Western society is about 10 per cent, with the corresponding figure for women being 4–5 per cent. The annual incidence figures for adults range between 0.2 and 0.7 per cent, so that each general practitioner may see about 12 new cases of peptic ulcer disease each year, in addition to having at least 100 patients with a history of peptic ulcer disease amongst the registered population.

The prevalence of GORD appears to be rising, for reasons that are not entirely clear. Peptic oesophagitis is now the most common abnormality found at endoscopy, and incidence and prevalence figures for this condition in general practice are increasing correspondingly. The majority of patients taking repeat prescriptions for acid-suppressing agents and antacids are likely to be receiving them for GORD rather than for peptic ulcer disease.

The incidence of malignant diseases of the upper gastrointestinal tract is much lower than that of peptic ulceration. In open-access endoscopy services, 1–2 per cent of all patients referred for investigation will be found to have overt malignancy, although more recent surveys, in which multiple biopsies are taken for histological examination, suggest that much greater numbers of patients have metaplastic and dysplastic changes which may represent pre-malignant states. These observations are discussed later, and are an important factor in determining the need for early investigation of patients with dyspeptic symptoms. The population incidence of oesophageal and gastric cancer is of the order of 20 per 100 000 per year, so that each general practitioner will probably see two new cases every three years or so. In the same way that a number of patients may have pre-malignant gastric lesions, a substantial proportion of patients with reflux symptoms and GORD will also develop the pre-malignant condition known as Barrett's oesophagus, in which the squamous lining of the lower oesophagus is replaced by metaplastic columnar epithelium. Adeno-carcinoma develops in Barrett's oesophagus at a rate of about 1 per 70 patient years, and the most appropriate arrangements for long-term surveillance of these patients by repeated endoscopy is currently a matter of considerable interest and debate.

LOWER GASTROINTESTINAL PROBLEMS

Symptoms in the community

Disorders of lower gastrointestinal function are, like those of the upper gastrointestinal tract, extremely common in the general population. A number of surveys have examined both the prevalence of colonic dysfunction and of rectal bleeding which, with abdominal pain, represent the three most frequently-reported symptoms, both by subjects studied in the community and by patients in general practitioners' surgeries.

A series of studies in North America and the UK have shown that colonic dysfunction is common in samples of apparently normal individuals who do not seek medical attention. A group in North Carolina, for example, have studied patients in the community and have found that 30–40 per cent of them report abdominal pain and disordered bowel function, with about 20 per cent of the general population meeting the diagnostic criteria for irritable bowel syndrome. In the UK researchers in Bristol have undertaken similar studies and have published broadly similar conclusions, that around 30–35 per cent of the general population reports a variety of abnormalities of colonic function, as well as abdominal pain, and about 20 per cent of the population also have features compatible with a clinical diagnosis of irritable bowel syndrome. The most recent population study from Southampton has confirmed these findings. In a carefully-selected random sample of more than 2000 patients, of whom more than 70 per cent returned a detailed questionnaire, 25 per cent of those replying had experienced more than six exposides of severe abdominal pain in preceding 12 months, and 22 per cent met the diagnostic criteria for irritable bowel syndrome (see Chapter 8 on functional bowel disorders). Diarrhoea and constipation were surprisingly common in the group as a whole, and occurred much more frequently in the subjects with irritable bowel syndrome. In the same way that only a minority of patients with upper gastrointestinal symptoms seek medical attention, so only about one-third of the patients with irritable bowel syndrome had consulted a general practitioner about their problems in the one-year study period.

In these and a number of other studies, the population prevalence of rectal bleeding has also been measured. Studies from the UK and Australia had previously reported one-year prevalence figures of rectal bleeding of between 12 and 18 per cent; in the Southampton survey, 20 per cent of the sample had experienced rectal bleeding, 15 per cent in the previous year. The prevalence was highest in subjects in the third and fourth decades of life, but even in late middle age, when the risk of colorectal cancer rises sharply, a prevalence figure of 10 per cent was found. Once again, only a small proportion of these patients with rectal bleeding had sought medical attention. In only one of these studies had the characteristics of rectal bleeding been investigated in detail; the majority of patients reporting bleeding had noticed blood on the toilet paper only, with only one per cent of the sample saying that the blood was mixed in with the stools. However Dent's study from Australia showed that the percentage of subjects reporting mixed blood depended on whether people examined their stools after defecation, with the figure for mixed bleeding rising to over 3 per cent in patients who inspected their stools more than half of the time.

Clinical conditions related to lower gastrointestinal symptoms

The clinical correlates of disordered bowel function and rectal bleeding are principally irritable bowel syndrome, diverticular disease (a rare cause of light rectal bleeding), inflammatory bowel disease, colorectal cancer, and perianal problems, such as haemorrhoids and anal fissures. This last group probably represents the most frequent explanation for rectal bleeding, although little encounter data is available for patients seen in general practice. The incidence of colorectal cancer in the population is, however, known with reasonable certainty and is approximately 40 per 100 000 per year. This means that the 'average' general practitioner with a list of around 2000 patients will see at least one if not two cases of colorectal cancer annually. The incidence of inflammatory bowel disease is much lower, with ulcerative colitis and Crohn's disease together accounting for 10 cases per 100 000 per year. This means that general practitioners may not see a new case of inflammatory bowel disease more than once every two to three years; the rarity of these conditions in primary care probably accounts for the well-documented delay in making a positive diagnosis, particularly when symptoms are mild and atypical. Several months or even years may pass before the diagnosis is made, partly because the symptoms reported by patients to general practitioners are much more likely to represent minor and self-limiting conditions. The triggers to investigation and referral are increasing frequency and severity of these symptoms.

CONSULTATION BEHAVIOUR

Most people with health problems do not seek medical advice from doctors. Diary studies in Europe and North America have shown that only about 1 in 40 symptoms becomes the subject of a medical encounter. The population surveys of upper and lower abdominal symptoms described above are consistent in their finding that only a minority—between one-quarter and one-third—of subjects consult general practitioners, with the remainder looking after their problems themselves, with support from family, social, and non-medical networks. What are the factors associated with consultation for gastrointestinal problems?

In considering questions of this kind it is most important to distinguish between *illness onset* and *illness declaration*; the first refers to the effect of personal, psychological, and physical factors in the production of symptoms or diseases, and the second to the factors which determine whether or not a person becomes a patient. The contribution of physical, social, and psychological factors in producing disorders such as peptic ulcer and irritable bowel syndrome are considered in other chapters of this book; the factors influencing illness declaration are dealt with here. In two detailed interview studies of subjects identified in population surveys with dyspepsia and with irritable bowel syndrome, who either had or had not consulted a general practitioner, symptom severity and frequency were not found to be the major determinants of consultation behaviour. Amongst the patients with dyspepsia, for example, the prevalence of quite severe and frequent symptoms among the non-consulting subjects and of relatively minor and infrequent symptoms amongst the consulters was striking. In patients with irritable bowel syndrome, symptom severity was of greater importance, with more pain being experienced by those who consulted general practitioners. This is in keeping with a recent study from Bristol which concluded that consulting patients with irritable bowel syndrome experienced more pain and more disruption of bowel function than control subjects who did not seek medical advice. In another study by a group from the Mayo clinic, symptom severity was found to account for only 25 per cent of the 'log likelihood' of consultation. Of much greater importance in both groups of patients are the health beliefs and concerns about the symptoms themselves. Amongst the dyspepsia patients fear of a serious or potentially fatal condition, of heart disease and of cancer were much more commonly seen amongst the patients who consulted general practitioners. This was also found in the irritable bowel syndrome patients, in whom abnormal scores on the Hospital Anxiety and Depression inventory were recorded, as well as more concern about serious illness and cancer, in the consulting group. In addition to these factors, recent experience of disruptive life events was also more frequent in the consulting group.

Of additional interest was the consistent finding in the dyspepsia and irritable bowel syndrome studies of the importance of the relationship between patients and individual general practitioners. In these studies patients with similar symptoms were found to consult at widely differing rates with different general practitioners. Amongst eight of these general practitioners, who had personal lists of patients, there was an order of magnitude difference between the lowest and highest consultation rates, suggesting that individual practitioners provide, whether consciously or not, reinforcement or deterrence for consultation with common symptoms, which influences their patients' consultation behaviour.

CLINICAL EPIDEMIOLOGY AND CLINICAL DECISION MAKING

General practitioners, as well as patients, vary considerably in their response to the common symptoms presented to them. In studies from Southampton, wide variations in the use of investigations, in referral rates to hospital out-patient clinics, and in prescribing rates and costs were observed amongst a large group of 179 general practitioners working in the same health district. Explanations for these differences could not be found when the characteristics of individual general practitioners, their workload, and the characteristics of their practices were correlated with use of resources, nor was there any consistent, systematic relationship between rates of, for example, prescribing and referral and use of investigations. The influences on general practitioners' clinical decision making are of considerable importance, particularly at a time of shrinking resources and when general practitioners are increasingly being given and seeking opportunities to manage their own budgets. One area of potentially productive research has been the investigation of general practitioners' estimates of risk and of their abilities to tolerate diagnostic uncertainty. For example, a study of general practitioners showed that there was a wide range in their estimates of the proportion of patients presenting with dyspeptic symptoms in whom subsequent investigation would reveal a significant organic lesion (peptic ulcer or cancer); estimates varied from 2 to 40 per cent of patients seen. The 'correct' answer is probably nearer 5 per cent, and wide deviation from this estimate is likely to be reflected in general practitioners' propensity to investigate or refer patients for specialist opinions. In studies on hypothetical clinical situations using vignettes of clinical cases, similar wide variation was seen in general practitioners' beliefs about the importance of undertaking investigations before beginning treatment. Even in cases in which the clinical history was strongly suggestive of a minor, diet-related gastrointestinal upset, a proportion of general practitioners opted for investigation before treatment; conversely in a scenario constructed to depict a typical high-risk patient with dyspeptic symptoms, a significant minority of general practitioners were prepared to treat empirically without obtaining a definitive endoscopic diagnosis. Further work is needed to tease out the factors, many of which have considerable relevance to continuing medical education, that appear to impact so strongly on decisions which have major resource and clinical consequences.

Of equal importance in considering the management of common conditions in primary care are the characteristics of investigations and tests used both in diagnosis and screening. General practitioners work in conditions of relatively low disease prevalence, while in hospital out-patient clinics investigations are chosen and ordered under conditions of much higher prevalence of 'serious' conditions. The characteristics of diagnostic tests vary according to the prevalence of the condition under test. Although the sensitivity (the proportion of patients with the target disorder who have a positive test result) and specificity (the proportion of patients without the disease who test negative) are virtually stable properties of diagnostic and screening tests, the positive and negative predictive values of these tests (the percentage of patients with positive or negative tests who, respectively, have or do not have the target disorder) vary according to the prevalence of the condition in the population under test. These considerations are important when thinking about the use of diagnostic tests, such as endoscopy and contrast radiology, and screening tests, such a faecal occult blood testing for colorectal neoplasia.

Interestingly, despite the disadvantages of working with ill-defined groups of symptoms in conditions of low disease prevalence, general practitioners appear to be remarkably good at selecting patients for investigation. A number of surveys of the use of barium meals, upper gastrointestinal endoscopy, and colonoscopy have shown that general practitioners' results, in terms of picking up significant lesions, are just as good as those obtained by their hospital colleagues. This is, perhaps, one of the strongest arguments for making investigations of this kind available on an open-access basis for general practitioners. The ability to obtain a rapid diagnosis without consultant referral is desirable for many patients because it saves time and resources. Anxieties about providing full access to investigations include possible confusion between a diagnostic test result and a specialist opinion, and the possibility that the referring doctor will not look beyond a negative test in patients with persistent symptoms which may have a basis in some other, serious organic problem. Concerns about increasing pressure on resources are also frequency articulated, although many physicians providing open-access encoscopy services claim that the increase in endoscopy time is more than balanced by savings in time in the out-patient clinic where, after all, up to one third of patients are referred for dyspeptic symptoms.

THE HOSPITAL INTERFACE

The wide variations in general practitioners' behaviour, particularly in relation to referral and use of investigations, suggests that guide-lines for good clinical practice, agreed between general practitioners and specialists might be useful. This almost certainly happens informally in a variety of ways; for example, endoscopists may stipulate that patients should be taken off ulcer-healing drugs before they are examined, so that the significance of the endoscopic findings is unequivocal. It is commonplace for radiology departments to insist on a sigmoidoscopy before a barium enema is performed, so that low colorectal lesions can be identified directly. It might, for example, be appropriate for hospitals to offer 'fast-track' access to sigmoidoscopy under these circumstances. Formal research evidence that guide-lines generated by general practitioners and hospital doctors are effective is, however, thin. In a large-scale study in Southampton, for example, a rather laboriously-generated set of guide-lines, circulated throughout the health district and evaluated in a randomized controlled trial produced only marginal effects on patterns of referral and investigation, although there was a significant increase in prescribing costs, principally of ulcer-healing agents. More research is needed in this area, particularly in relation to appropriate investigation and early detection of significant problems, such as inflammatory bowel disease and cancer. Some endoscopy units, for example, provide full open-access, with no restriction on general practitioners' use of the service, although a recent national survey has shown that the majority of so-called open-access services actually involve some kind of 'vetting' of endoscopy requests by specialists. The possibility that full open-access endoscopy might lead to earlier detection of oesophageal and gastric cancer was initially discounted in studies in Southampton and Bournemouth, but more recent work in Birmingham, for example, suggests that early gastric cancer might well be detected more frequently if investigation was carried out on dyspeptic patients at an earlier stage. Other endoscopy units provide formal request cards, sometimes incorporating a scoring system based on history and clinical features, so that general practitioners can only order the investigation if patients meet certain pre-determined criteria. It may well be that such hospital-led guidelines, which are likely to be informed by current research evidence, provide a more realistic way of influencing the use of resources. There are real difficulties in modifying individual general practitioner's behaviour; many instances of mis-diagnosis and diagnostic delay can be traced to sub-optimal clinical assessment and management, and it is unlikely that major improvements can be achieved simply by circulating documents from hospital units.

It is important to remember, in relation to the interface between general practice and the hospital, that many general practitioners work as clinical assistants or hospital practitioners in gastroenterology units, generally doing endoscopies. A recent national survey showed that about 160 general practitioners are involved in this kind of work, providing an average of 1.5 clinical sessions per week in the majority of district general hospital endoscopy units. These general practitioners provide a highly-trained and stable pool of expertise, in contrast to rapidly-changing junior medical staff, and are a valuable resource as well as an important link between the worlds of hospital medicine and primary care. Unfortunately, there is also evidence that the new contract for general practitioners has made many of these doctors re-evaluate their role in the hospital, largely because the terms of service and remuneration for providing these sessions are relatively poor.

PRESCRIBING

The level of prescribing for gastrointestinal disorders is increasing, both in price and volume, and represents a very significant proportion of the total drug budget in the UK. The number of prescriptions dispensed in the gastrointestinal group from the *British National Formulary* (BNF) in 1979 was 27 million, rising to 33 million in 1989, making gastrointestinal prescribing the sixth highest group in terms of volume. The average net ingredient cost per prescription has risen even more sharply, from £2.06 in 1979 to £8.61 in 1989. The average net ingredient cost of gastrointestinal drugs ranked third in 1989 behind dressings and appliances and rheumatic preparations. Prescriptions for ulcer-healing agents represent a substantial proportion of these costs, which are likely to rise as newer agents to treat acid-related disorders and dysmotility become available.

The enormous cost consequences of prescribing make it more important than ever that general practitioners and hospital doctors are aware not only of the efficacy, safety, and acceptability of the drugs they prescribe, but also of their cost. The Prescription Pricing Authority now provides regular Prescribing Analysis and Cost (PACT) information about prescribing costs and patterns, each practice has now been given an indicative prescribing amount, regulated through each FHSA, and Medical Advisers are now employed by all FHSAs to advise on good prescribing practices. Many of these developments represent mechanisms for producing downward pressure on prescribing; unfortunately much of the research evidence on which to base statements about 'good' practice is simply unavailable. Many factors may influence practice prescribing, including changes in list size, demographic patterns, and changes in balance of care and prescribing between hospitals and general practice. Additionally, screening and surveillance programmes and audit activities are likely to identify previously unrecognized or unmet health needs, and may well lead to higher prescribing rates and costs. This is certainly true of conditions such as asthma, and it may well be true for a variety of gastrointestinal problems.

This will be a continuing issue for discussion, irrespective of the political or economic shape of the National Health Service of the future. We know quite a lot about the structure and process of care in prescribing, but much less about outcome. Our understanding and ability to measure health needs in populations and the health status of groups of patients is often poor; general practice desperately needs many of the skills of clinical epidemiology to make measurements of this kind. Outcome measures remain crude, with Standardised Mortality Rates being the most frequently-used index of the health status of communities. The ability to measure quality of life and functional status, and accurately to monitor changes in these parameters, both in individuals and in populations, is needed before we are able to make confident statements about the value of prescribing, or other medical interventions.

AUDIT

The regular and accurate collection and review of data in general practice is now part of our terms and conditions of service, and FHSAs and Regional Health Authorities also have a statutory obligation to show that clinical work in primary care is the subject of audit. Although gastro-intestinal disorders are much less popular targets for audit than, for example, hypertension and diabetes, a number of aspects of the clinical care of gastrointestinal conditions are appropriate audit topics. Repeat prescription of ulcer-healing drugs, which represent a very substantial part of the drug budget, is one area in which practices might consider review. Criteria for comparison might include the recording of a confirmed diagnosis before long-term therapy was started, the adequacy of symptom relief, the frequency of relapses in patients with duodenal ulcer (possible need for other forms of therapy) and the duration of symptoms in patients with gastro-oesophageal reflux disease (possible need for endoscopic review).

In relation to lower gastrointestinal problems, similar examples might include faecal occult blood screening in patients with positive family histories or other risk factors for colorectal cancer, adequacy or surveillance and follow-up of patients with inflammatory bowel disease, and symptom control (possible need for referral or other therapy) in patients with functional bowel disorders. One audit-related approach to promoting good clinical care of gastrointestinal problems in general practice might be the development of guide-lines by local Medical Audit Advisory Groups (MAAGs). For example it might be appropriate for MAAGs to make recommendations about the desirable level of investigation (proctoscopy, sigmoidoscopy, etc.) in general practice, or to enable rates of prescribing and investigation for gastrointestinal disorders to be reviewed and compared with similar data from local practices serving similar populations.

Audit should not be seen as solely based in general practice, however; information obtained from the audit of any condition may have significance for the provision of hospital facilities and this is particularly true for gastrointestinal problems. Difficulties in obtaining investigations, for example, may be reflected in other features of clinical care, and MAAGs may be able to comment on inadequacies of this kind to provider units.

RESEARCH

General practice offers enormous opportunities for research in gastro-intestinal disorders. The natural history of many of the common conditions with which we are faced still remains uncertain, and cohorts of patients can be identified and followed in general practice, providing a perspective of their illness which more accurately reflects the community and primary care settings in which they are managed. A major national study on the efficacy of colorectal cancer screening will report in the near future; general practitioners are probably best placed to offer screening of this kind, and research on the most effective strategies for assuring compliance is of importance if it is shown that mortality can be reduced in this way. Selection of patients for investigation and identification of those at high risk of serious disease is, once again, something that can best be undertaken in general practice. Information of this kind, collected in the hospital out-patients setting, is rarely representative of the range of problems seen by general practitioners; accurate definition of the clinical characteristics of patients who turn out to have unexpected serious disorders, particularly gastrointestinal malignancies, is of considerable importance. There is, for example, a pressing need to develop a better understanding of the natural history of patients presenting with rectal bleeding, in whom accurate selection for early investigation of inflammatory and malignant lesions is crucial, but at present is carried out in a less than satisfactory way.

FURTHER READING

Dent, O. F., Goulston, K. J., Zurbrzycki, J., and Chapuis, P. H. (1986). Bowel symptoms in an apparently well population. *Diseases of the Colon and Rectum*, **29**, 243–7.

Drossman, D. A., Sandler, R. S., McKee, D. C., and Lovitz, A. J. (1982). Bowel patterns among subjects not seeking health care. *Gastroenterology*, **83**, 529–34.

Heaton, K. W., Ghosh, S., and Braddon, F. E.M. (1991). How bad are the symptoms and bowel dysfunction of patients with the irritable bowel syndrome? *Gut*, **32**, 73–9.

Jones, R. (1987). Self-care and primary care of dyspepsia: a review. *Family Practice*, **4**, 68–77.

Jones, R. H., Lydeard, S. E., Hobbs, F. D. R., Kenkre, J. E., Williams, E. I., Repper, J. A., *et al*. (1990). Dyspepsia in England and Scotland. *Gut*, **31**, 401–5.

Jones, R. and Lydeard, S. (1992). Irritable bowel syndrome in the general population. *British Medical Journal*, **304**, 87–90.

Kettell, J., Jones, R., and Lydeard, S. (1992). Reasons for consultation in irritable bowel syndrome: symptoms and patients characteristics. *British Journal of General Practice*, **42**, 459–61.

Lydeard, S., Jones, R. (1989). Factors affecting the decision to consult with dyspepsia: comparison of consulters and non-consulters. *Journal of the Royal College of General Practitioners*, **39**, 495–8.

2 Investigating the gastro-intestinal tract

Pali Hungin and Michael Bramble

During the last decade there has been a change in the role of the general practitioner in the management of gastrointestinal problems, especially dyspepsia. The major contributory factors have been advances in drug therapy and wider availability of accurate investigations, in particular endoscopy. The narrowing of the gap between general practitioners and specialists with regard to patient management has meant that, perhaps more than in any other field, the general practitioner has gained ground in terms of comprehensive patient care.

AVAILABILITY AND ACCESS TO INVESTIGATIONS

The extent to which a general practitioner is able to manage the patient is dependent on the accessibility of local investigative services, as well as facilities within the practice for on-site procedures. There are still wide discrepancies in the availability of open-access facilities for general practitioners, with variations not only between regions but also between different health authorities in the same region. However, controversies and decisions previously deferred are now being driven by the changes in the National Health Service, with the purchaser-provider split providing new impetus for seeking easier access to hospital-based facilities.

Open-access gastroscopy

Most specialists agree that open-access gastroscopy should be provided, but there is disagreement as to whether it should be on the basis of true open-access, i.e. without prior reference to the specialist, or on a 'censored' basis where the general practitioner is required to contact the specialist first. The British Society of Gastroenterology stated in its 1990 report *Provision of gastrointestinal endoscopy* that open-access endoscopy should be provided by all endoscopy units, albeit with concurrent educational initiatives for general practitioners, and the possibility of scrutiny of requests.

Contrary to traditional fears, providing open-access does not result in swamping of the local service, and there is evidence that the total hospital workload actually drops. There is an associated reduction in barium meal examination requests by general practitioners, and a low secondary referral rate following the gastroscopy. The importance of a normal gastroscopy result is increasingly recognized as part of the overall management of the patient, and there is evidence to suggest that this may also be associated with a reduction in gastrointestinal prescribing and consultation rates.

It should be noted, however, that the impact of open-access gastroscopy is dependent on a short waiting time, and local arrangements, including a degree of screening, may be necessary to maintain an effective service.

Open-access barium enema

As for gastroscopy there are inconsistencies in the availability of open-access barium enema within and between Regions. Some radiologists have been reluctant to offer this service unless a sigmoidscopy was performed first to exclude recto-sigmoid lesions. There are also increasing fears about the level of radiation exposure during an examination, enhancing the need for an appropriate indication for the procedure. This must be balanced against an increasing awareness about colonic polyps and the need for the early detection of colonic cancer.

Open-access sigmoidscopy

Some centres offer an open-access rigid sigmoidscopy service, sometimes allied to a radiology department offering barium enemas. The concept of open-access flexible (fibre-optic) sigmoidscopy is gaining credence, particularly in light of the pressures for an early and accurate diagnosis for patients with rectal bleeding. There are little data on the likely overall demand if such a service were available nationally, but many gastro-enterologists are willing to provide a limited service to general practitioners who contact them.

Open-access cholecystography and ultrasound scanning

Although cholecystography is generally available on open-access, ultrasound scanning is only patchily provided, even though it offers several clinical advantages and does not necessarily require the services of a radiologist.

THE OESOPHAGUS, STOMACH, AND DUODENUM

Barium meal

At the time of writing the barium meal is still the most common upper gastrointestinal investigation ordered by general practitioners.

Advantages and indications

The chief advantage of a barium meal is that it is non-invasive, virtually nationally available on open-access, and offers a convenient method of visualizing the upper gastrointestinal tract. Oesophageal motility can be assessed by studying the wave forms of barium transit in disorders which affect the oesophageal body as well as the lower oesophageal spincter. Pharyngeal pouches, cervical webs, and oesophageal diverticulae and hiatus herniae are well demonstrated.

The investigation is particularly indicated where an oesophageal lesion is suspected, as an investigation of dysphagia prior to gastroscopy, and for the detection and assessment of gastro-oesophageal reflux and hiatus hernia. Where an oesophageal study is specifically required, a barium swallow is more appropriate (see below).

Shortcomings

Although much improved by the use of a double contrast barium technique the radiological diagnosis of mucosal disease is controversial, and acute gastritis, erosions, and chronic gastritis are not associated with characteristic features. The diagnosis of atrophic gastritis also cannot be made with certainty and a duodenal ulcer may be missed against the backdrop of a scarred cap. In practical terms barium meal examinations may miss a significant proportion of peptic ulcers and gastric carcinomata whilst also giving a significant number of false positives. The overall detection rate of lesions is around 25 per cent, and for dyspepsia sensitivity and specificity rates of 34 per cent and 91 per cent respectively have been reported.

Hiatus herniae are liable to being overdiagnosed because of confusion with normal lower distal oesophageal distension and different demonstration techniques used by radiologists.

Pylorospasm may occur as a result of patient anxiety, although it can indicate organic disease at the gastric outlet. Where chronic outlet obstruction exists, barium retention can interfere with an effective examination of the stomach.

In addition, the risks associated with radiation exposure need to be considered, and a barium meal is contraindicated in pregnancy.

The procedure

A double contrast examination involves swallowing about 200 ml of barium sulphate suspension together with a gas-producing agent, usually an effervescent tablet. The patient normally fasts for 5 hours prior to the examination and may be given a drug (for example, intravenous glucagon), to produce transient gastric atony. The patient usually lies on a mechanized table which moves in different planes allowing the contrast medium to coat the entire luminal lining. Image intensification, and video monitoring and recording techniques may also be used.

In order to demonstrate a hiatus hernia and gastro-oesophageal reflux the patient may require tilting in the prone position combined with the application of pressure over the abdomen, and may be asked to perform various swallowing manoeuvres in addition to coughing, straining, and leg raising. Free gastro-oesophageal reflux of contrast is considered significant and the presence of a stricture or ulceration at a level higher than the gastro-oesophageal junction may indicate Barrett's oesophagus or cancer. The rate of gastric emptying can be used as a measure of vagotomy success and as an aid to the diagnosis of dumping.

Barium meal examinations are generally very well tolerated. However, because of the effort required in swallowing the contrast medium and the effervescent tablets, and the positioning requirements to obtain satisfactory views, barium meal examinations are not, contrary to belief, necessarily well or easily performed in the frail or the elderly. Diabetic patients may also present problems because of the need to fast before the examination. This applies especially to insulin controlled diabetics, and close liaison between the radiologist and the general practitioner requesting the procedure is essential.

Barium swallow

Radiological examination of the oesophagus should now be regarded as a test separate from the conventional barium meal. The development of techniques for demonstrating oesophageal problems has led to several variations of the traditional barium swallow. These include swallowing radiolabelled particles of food in order to observe and to identify specific areas of obstruction and dysmotility of the oesophagus. In expert hands, with the use of labelled 'bread' or 'marshmallow' swallows detailed functional studies can be performed.

Gastroscopy

Gastroscopy is well established in the investigation of haematemesis, dyspepsia, and other abdominal symptoms. Developments in fibre-optic and image processing technology mean that modern instruments are considerably slimmer, with greater manoeuvrability. The image can be conveyed directly on to a colour monitor with facilities for video recording and photography. In addition to being a diagnostic tool the endoscope can be used for a variety of impressive therapeutic procedures, including oesophageal dilatation, injection sclerotherapy of bleeding ulcers and oesophageal varices, and the laser treatment of bleeding ulcers and tumours. Secondary diagnostic procedures using contrast media injected via the endoscope can also be performed.

Gastroscopy is used for visualization of the oesophagus, stomach, pylorus, and duodenum. Biopsies and scraped cytology specimens can be obtained for suspected mucosal inflammation, peptic ulceration, carcinoma, *Helicobacter* gastritis, and adult coeliac disease. Histological specimens are routinely used in some centres for detecting the presence of *Helicobacter pylori* by means of a urease test, a relatively simple side-room procedure.

Gastroscopes vary in the angle of vision available and as to whether they are forward, side, or oblique viewing. The most commonly used diagnostic instrument is forward viewing, and measures approximately 12 mm in diameter. Accompanying equipment consists of a quartz halogen light source and suction and air insufflation equipment to allow the endoscopist to reduce or distend the lumen. The endoscopist requires the assistance of at least one specially trained nurse.

Preparation for gastroscopy

Prior to the examination the patient is required to have taken no solids for at least six hours. No liquids are taken for four hours. For many procedures topical pharyngeal anaesthesia is sufficient and is accomplished with the use of a lignocaine spray. In some instances, especially in the anxious patient, intravenous sedation is used. This is usually Diazemuls (a modified diazepam formulation) which has a rapid onset sedative action. Intravenous hyoscine may also be necessary to produce gastric paresis in order to obtain a better view. This produces a dry mouth as a side-effect. The intravenous sedation commonly results in amnesia for the examination itself. Patients should have the choice of selecting their preferred pre-gastroscopy medication, but intravenous sedation does have disadvantages, in that the patient is not allowed to return home unaccompanied, or to drive or operate machinery for 48 hours afterwards.

The procedure

A plastic tooth-guard is inserted between the teeth and the instrument is introduced into the oesophagus by guiding the angulated flexible tip. The average time for a straightforward diagnostic gastroscopy is generally no more than 5 minutes. The patient is usually examined in the left lateral position. Biopsy and cytology scrapings are taken by introducing cabled forceps and brushes through channels in the instrument. At all times only gentle pressure is involved in advancing the instrument and, indeed, undue resistance can indicate an obstructive lesion. For this reason oesophageal examination requires great care, particularly if a stricture or neoplasm is suspected.

Tolerability, safety, and problems

Diagnostic gastroscopy is surprisingly well tolerated, with intubation failure being comparatively rare (1–2 per cent). Providing no therapeutic manoeuvre, such as oesophageal dilatation, is being attempted gastroscopy can be considered safe. The trachea is occasionally inadvertently entered, resulting in a fit of coughing or temporary laryngeal spasm. Minor aspiration pneumonitis occurs rarely. To date the most common complications quoted are local reactions at the intravenous injection site, but these, too, have declined with the change from diazepam to Diazemuls for sedation. Oesophageal perforation remains a serious complication, but the incidence is extremely low for diagnostic gastroscopy. Mortality rates of 0.02 per cent or 1 in 4400 have been quoted, but these included procedures in which therapeutic intervention was being attempted, for example the treatment of bleeding ulcers. Respiratory depression and cardiac arrest are potential problems and vigilance with patients with respiratory or cardiovascular disease is necessary.

Gastroscopy is surprisingly well tolerated by the elderly, although close care is required in case of respiratory and cardiovascular complications. Most endoscopy units now use continuous pulse and tissue oxygen saturation devices thoughout the procedure.

How accurate is gastroscopy?

Gastroscopy has been the gold standard for detection of lesions in the upper gastrointestinal tract for a long time, but the procedure is now being reassessed in terms of its accuracy. Variation between endoscopists, and problems with the definition and description of musocal morphology have caused obvious difficulties in terms of consistent conclusions. Whilst being the best investigation available, with a quoted sensitivity of 92 per cent and specificity of 100 per cent for dyspeptic problems, mucosal lesions are notoriously difficult to categorize objectively and can be misreported. Differences between endoscopists in their grading of oesophagitis is common, and descriptions of redness or hyperaemia indicating inflammation are not reliable. A morphological diagnosis of antral oedema, gastritis, or duodenitis is subject to equal variation and even apparently confirmatory evidence from histology can be subject to similar inconsistencies. Indeed, the significance of many recorded mucosal changes in the stomach is not clinically clear in the light of present knowledge, even though these findings may be used to provide an explanation for some clinical symptomatology.

There is much greater accuracy in the reporting of lesions breaching the mucosa, for example, ulcers and cancers. Nonetheless, ulcers, particularly duodenal ulcers, are not infrequently missed, especially those lying behind a mucosal fold, and it should be remembered that lesions may have healed or be in remission by the time the patient has the gastroscopy. The presence or absence of gastro-oesophageal reflux and the diagnosis of hiatus hernia cannot always be made with certainty, although serious oesophageal mucosal damage and varices are well recorded.

Recognition of the concept of non-ulcer dyspepsia has highlighted some of the shortcomings of gastroscopy as a means of reaching a definite confirmatory or exclusion diagnosis, but has also offered a means of further investigation, for example, for the presence of *Helicobacter pylori* infection. It needs to be noted there is not always an undeniable link between clinical symptomatology and gastroscopy findings, and the investigation should not be seen as a means to an end in itself.

Gastroscopy or barium meal?

Following a long period of controversy it is now generally accepted that gastroscopy is the preferable investigation except in certain specific instances. The overall detection rate of lesions using barium meals is around 25 per cent, compared with around 35 per cent for gastroscopy, excluding the detection of *Helicobacter pylori* infection. One of the indications for gastroscopy remains the follow-up of a doubtful or negative barium meal examination.

In the investigation of dyspepsia, endoscopy has been shown to be more sensitive (92 per cent versus 34 per cent) and specific (100 per cent versus 91 per cent) than the double contrast barium meal. Gastroscopy also has the advantage of allowing histological and cytological specimens to be taken, as well as detecting *Helicobacter pylori* infection.

In terms of patient tolerance, contrary to popular belief, endoscopy may be the easier choice for most patients. It is a short procedure with a relatively low level of discomfort. It is quicker than a barium meal examination and the patient does not need to be tilted or rotated, and manoeuvres to increase intra-abdominal pressure to demonstrate reflux and a hiatus hernia are not necessary. In the elderly and frail a barium meal may involve greater discomfort, and in the event of an equivocal result the gastroscopy may be required anyway.

The value of a barium study lies in the investigation of the oesophagus and the gastro-oesophageal junction. A study of the flow of barium through the oesophagus is a useful technique for observing motility and the site of a lesion. With the use of specialized swallowing techniques involving labelled 'swallows' it is possible to link the oesophageal transit problems with presenting symptomatology. However, where there is an indication of pathology other than uncomplicated oesophagitis, or where the reflux appears clinically severe, endoscopy is the procedure of choice. These include patients whose initial symptoms are dysphagia (where a barium swallow is likely to be done prior to gastroscopy), progressive symptoms despite therapy, or a patient with a previous history of an obstructive oesophageal lesion. Severe reflux oesophagitis and malignancy need early specific diagnosis for effective therapy, and histological assessment is important.

In patients in whom radiology has indicated a duodenal ulcer as the sole lesion, gastroscopy is not required unless the response to therapy is poor, in which case alternative lesions have to be excluded. If the radiological findings are normal or equivocal, endoscopy may be helpful for a precise diagnosis, for example, in a report of cap deformity or spasm. However, endoscopy is not necessary for the follow-up of a duodenal ulcer noted on a previous barium meal, although it is indicated for gastric ulcers.

Twenty-four hour intra-oesophageal pH monitoring

The procedure

This is a relatively new technique, now available in many hospitals, in which an antimony or glass electrode is used to record intra-oesophageal pH and a solid-state recorder to store collected data. A relatively inexpensive desktop computer is used to analyse the results. The procedure involves passing the electrode via the nose into the upper oesophagus and then positioning it at a distance of 5 cm above the gastro-oesophageal junction as previously determined by manometry or gastro-scopy. Fluoroscopy may sometimes be used to confirm its position. The antimony electrode is the smallest available and sits at the end of a fine-bore tube measuring 2–3 mm in diameter. The electrode is secured in position and the recorder strapped to the patient's waist using a belt and holster arrangement.

The patient is then allowed to return home and encouraged to have a normal day apart from being required to fill in a detailed diary card indicating times of meals, times when supine and also to note episodes of chest pain or heartburn. There is also usually a button on the solid-state recorder which can be depressed if the patient experiences symptoms and this will leave a permanent record on the trace. The patient returns 24 hours later to have the pH probe removed. Data from the recorder is downloaded into the computer, which analyses the trace producing a graphic summary of intra-oesophageal pH during the 24-hour period. It is also possible to correlate this with episodes of chest pain or heartburn.

Indications

Twenty-four hour intra-oesophageal pH monitoring is usually not indicated for patients who are known to have endoscopically proven oesophagitis. The test is much more useful in confirming gastro-oesophageal reflux as a cause for patients' symptoms where the endoscopy is normal, or where there is some doubt regarding the aetiology of chest pain. To some extent it has become the gold standard for measuring gastro-oesophageal reflux disease (GORD) and has largely replaced the Bernstein test.

Oesophageal manometry

The procedure

Oesophageal manometry refers to tests carried out in hospital which measure lower oesophageal sphincter pressure and intra-oesophageal pressure changes in response to swallowing. The strength and duration of contractions are recorded as well as the number of peristaltic and non-peristaltic swallows. There is also an important function for oesophageal manometry in diagnosing achalasia of the cardia, which is characterized by the lower oesophageal sphincter failing to relax on swallowing. Oesophageal manometry is not widely used, but is available in most teaching centres.

A fine-bore multi-lumen tube is passed into the oesophagus via the nasal route and perfused continuously with water. The pressure changes are measured using transducers, which then relay the information to a recorder and printer, producing a graphic printout of the results. This investigation is also made a good deal easier by the use of a desktop microcomputer.

Indications

The main indication for oesophageal manometry is the further investigation of non-obstructive dysphagia or atypical chest pain.

SMALL INTESTINE

Barium meal follow-through and small bowel enema

These investigations are indicated where malabsorption, inflammatory bowel disease, or unexplained abdominal pain merits investigation.

The barium mixture can be taken orally and the examination performed as a follow-up of a conventional barium meal. If a specific demonstration of part of the small intestine is required the barium is delivered directly into the jejunum with a tube passed orally through to the duodenum. This latter method, a small bowel enema, is also useful if problems with gastric outflow obstruction are anticipated.

Small bowel enema

For this procedure the throat is anaesthetized topically and intubation performed using a guide-wire passed through to the duodenum. As well as observing the passage of the barium through the small intestine, X-rays can be taken at specific points, or the images stored on videotape. Following intubation the investigation usually takes only minutes when the upper part of the small intestine is being studied. This procedure is particularly useful for aiding the diagnosis of sub-acute obstruction.

In some instances the terminal ileum is better demonstrated by a barium enema.

Barium meal follow-through

This is performed less frequently now. Its function is to demonstrate the small bowel, from the jejunum to the ileo-caecal junction. The examination is a lengthy one, sometimes lasting more than 24 hours. Although the patient may be allowed to eat after the proximal small intestine has been outlined the examination requires a degree of perseverance. Pro-kinetic drugs may be used to accelerate the passage of the barium and X-rays are taken at intervals, initially every 15 minutes. Exposure to radiation is greater than in a small bowel enema, and the results are less satisfactory.

This investigation can help in the diagnosis of malabsorption syndromes by indicating reduced transit time, ileal distension or stricture, and thickening of intestinal folds. With the use of a non-flocculating barium suspension Crohn's disease, strictures, diverticulae, and blind loops can also be demonstrated.

THE GALL-BLADDER, BILE DUCTS, AND PANCREAS

Plain abdominal X-ray

Up to 20 per cent of gallstones can be seen on a plain abdominal X-ray. Calcium-containing stones are radio-opaque, but pure cholesterol stones are radiolucent.

Oral cholecystography

This is the most common investigation of the gall-bladder. It is available virtually nationally on open-access and requires very little radiography time.

The procedure

The patient needs to be on a fat-free diet for the day before the examination and to take about six contrast medium tablets with the evening meal on the day before the examination. These can cause nausea and vomiting. The contrast medium is excreted by the liver, concentrated in the gall-bladder, and expelled via the bile duct.

X-ray films are taken in the erect and horizontal postures and computerized tomography is performed in cases of poor visualization of the gall-bladder. Gall-bladder stimulation is then produced, either by a fatty meal or a pre-prepared fatty drink, or occasionally with the use of an injection of cholecystokinin. Thereafter films are taken at 20–60 minute intervals.

Disadvantages

A drawback of oral cholecystography is that the cystic duct is not demonstrated in some instances and the common bile duct is only occasionally outlined. Also, failure of gall-bladder contraction does not necessarily indicate disease, and the examination may need to be repeated with a higher dose of contrast medium and films at longer intervals. It is not as useful as ultrasound scanning in acute cholecystitis, where cystic duct obstruction occurs.

Accuracy

With a careful technique, oral cholecystography is highly accurate (95–99 per cent accuracy), with positive evidence of 70 per cent and presumptive evidence of 98 per cent of gallstones and up to 95 per cent of significant cholecystitis. Gallstones as small as 1–2 mm can be visualized. It should be noted, however, that in a patient with a non-functioning gall-bladder, or in the presence of obstructive jaundice, little or no information is obtained even if the patient has gallstones. Ultrasound scanning should be performed instead.

Ultrasound scanning of the upper abdomen

Indications and advantages

This is a popular, non-invasive, and safe method for investigating the gall-bladder and the common bile duct. In expert hands the method can be 98 per cent accurate for gallstones, especially those over 3 mm in diameter, and can be useful for demonstrating acute cholecystitis or a thickened gall-bladder wall. It also helps accurately to determine the size of the intrahepatic ducts and can show a mass in the pancreatic head. The equipment required for ultrasound scanning is relatively straightforward and the examination does not necessarily require a radiologist. The examination can be completed in minutes and offers an obvious advantage over the cholecystogram. It is useful especially in being able to locate the head of the pancreas, and it is usually possible to report on the kidneys and liver parenchyma. However, it cannot accurately differentiate between localized pancreatitis and carcinoma and is severely limited by the presence of intestinal gas.

The procedure

The preparation for an ultrasound scan of the gall-bladder and associated structures is similar to that for a barium meal. The patient is usually required to starve for five hours, usually by means of an overnight fast for a morning examination.

The technique uses a transducer producing a pulse of high-frequency sound waves. These ultrasound waves are reflected and refracted by intra-abdominal structures and the resulting echoes are converted into electrical impulses. A rapid transmission and echo detection sequence is produced and displayed on a visual display unit for still photography or video recording. Scanning requires the presence of a layer of gel between the transducer and the skin, and the resulting echoes are depicted in varying shades, allowing a decipherable picture to be completed. There is no patient discomfort.

Intravenous cholangiography

Intravenous cholangiography is used relatively infrequently now. It may be useful if duct pathology is suspected, in patients who have had a cholecystectomy, in the vomiting patient, or if the oral cholecystogram was unsuccessful. It may also help in an acute situation where the diagnosis needs to be established rapidly. The contrast medium used to be injected intravenously, but is now slowly infused by drip over a period of 10–30 minutes. Tomographic X-rays are taken after allowing 30 minutes for opacification of the intrahepatic ducts and the common bile duct. Providing the cystic duct is patent, gall-bladder opacification occurs, although this may take 6–24 hours. In acute cholecystitis the gall-bladder does not fill as the cystic duct is obstructed.

Even in patients with a normal serum bilirubin there is a failure to demonstrate the duct in about 6 per cent of patients and the success rate declines with an increase in bilirubin concentration. Intravenous cholangiography is generally well tolerated, although a serious reaction to the contrast medium remains a rare risk.

Percutaneous transhepatic cholangiography

The procedure

This procedure is carried out in the X-ray department under local (skin) anaesthesia.

A Skinny (Chiba) needle is passed into the liver through a tract anaesthetized using 2 per cent lignocaine. The needle is usually inserted through the ninth intercostal space in the mid-axillary line, but as the procedure is performed under X-ray screening control the operator may try a second approach if the first is unsuccessful. As the needle is withdrawn, small amounts of contrast medium are injected until a bile duct is entered and filled with contrast. At this point more dye is injected with the aim of completely filling the biliary tree. Radiographs are then taken to show the anatomy of the biliary tree and any abnormalities.

Indications

The main indication for this technique is the further investigation of obstructive jaundice or abnormal liver function tests and where endoscopic retrograde cholangio-pancreatography (ERCP) has failed. Therapeutic options include stent insertion for the palliative treatment of bile duct strictures and cholangiocarcinoma, as well as temporary decompression of the biliary tree using an internal/external drain.

The procedure can also be used to facilitate cannulation of the common bile duct at ERCP where previous attempts have failed. This dual approach increases the success rate of therapeutic ERCP and reduces further the number of patients requiring laparotomy.

Endoscopic retrograde cholangio-pancreatography (ERCP)

The procedure

ERCP refers to an examination of the biliary tree and pancreas by cannulating the ampulla of Vater and performing a retrograde injection of a radio-opaque dye into the pancreas and common bile duct. The procedure is carried out in the X-ray department, usually under intravenous sedation along similar lines to a gastroscopy, although the sedation tends to be more profound in order for the endoscopist to be able to cannulate the ampulla and obtain adequate pictures. A side-viewing endoscope is required for this procedure. There are two therapeutic options to ERCP, one of which necessitates a sphincterotomy (a small cut through the sphincter muscle made at the time of the procedure utilizing a diathermy current). Following sphincterotomy it is possible to extract stones from within the common bile duct by passing either a balloon catheter or a Dormier basket into the common bile duct and extracting the stone through the enlarged sphincterotomy.

The second therapeutic option for patients with obstructive jaundice who have a carcinoma of the pancreas or cholangiocarcinoma is to insert a stent (a hollow tube made of Teflon or similar material) into the common bile duct in order to open up the stricture and allow free drainage of bile into the duodenum. Stents placed across strictures in this way usually remain patent for approximately six months and can be replaced easily if drainage becomes inadequate due to 'silting up' of the prosthesis. Stent insertion requires the use of a large channel (4.2 mm) side-viewing endoscope.

Indications

The main indication for ERCP is the further investigation of obstructive jaundice. This usually follows on from an ultrasound scan of the biliary tree which has shown a dilated biliary system. Indications for stent insertion include obstructive jaundice in elderly patients or patients considered unfit for surgery. The procedure is now being used increasingly in younger patients who have inoperable malignant disease, as the results appear to be very similar to operative bypass surgery.

ERCP is also a very effective way of looking for pancreatic abnormalities, although not necessarily pancreatic carcinoma or pancreatic pseudocyst. In patients with suspected chronic pancreatitis abnormalities that are not evident on either ultrasound or computerized tomography (CT) scanning are usually detected by ERCP. ERCP is therefore a sensitive investigation of pancreatic anatomy which may demonstrate the earliest changes of chronic pancreatitis long before any other abnormalities can be detected.

Computerized tomographic (CT) scans

Indications and equipment

This technique enables cross-sectional imaging with clear definition of intra-abdominal structures, including the pancreas and biliary tree. The procedure is accurate and especially indicated for pancreatic lesions, although endoscopic ultrasound examinations are now also being used for this purpose. The camera uses sensitive X-ray detectors and a computer to extrapolate information from the level of absorption of the radiation. The device consists of a scanning unit with an X-ray source and an adjustable examination couch, together with ancillary equipment for imaging, data storage, and printing. A fan-shaped beam scans the patient at cuts of 13 mm through 180° plane, each section taking about 30 seconds. The images can be stored by the computer or printed as required.

The procedure

Before the examination, the patient is maintained on a low residue diet and multiple contrast media are usually utilized, especially if the target is the head of the pancreas. In some instances contrast media may need to be given by mouth and rectally, as well as intravenously.

CT scans are expensive and involve radiation exposure greater than in conventional radiology. The procedure can be an ordeal for the patient because of the concurrent use of contrast media, the level of preparation required, and the necessity to lie very still.

THE LOWER GASTROINTESTINAL TRACT

Digital rectal examination

The rectal examination is still part of good clinical practice in general practice. General practitioners are sometimes reluctant to subject the patient to a repeated examination if a referral to hospital is being made, but not all specialists are sympathetic to the consultation conditions in practice with regard to time, workload pressure, and lack of chaperoning assistance. A measure of the importance of the examination is that about 15 per cent of all bowel cancers can be felt digitally, even though in absolute terms this may be a rare event in the career of a general practitioner.

For a successful examination the patient should have an understanding of the need for the examination. With the patient in the left lateral position the buttocks are parted and the anus inspected. The right index finger, well lubricated, is inserted slowly. After noting the sphincteric tone the finger is swept around circumferentially, taking in the sacral curve and the lateral pelvic walls. Rectal polyps may be felt as soft masses and are sometimes mistaken for faeces. Internal haemorrhoids are felt only if they are thrombosed or very large and a neoplastic growth usually presents as an indurated ulcerating lesion or as a narrowing of the lumen.

Proctoscopy

This examination is well within the range of the general practitioner. It is a good method for diagnosing internal haemorrhoids as well as fissures, fistulae, and low rectal cancers. However, a false sense of security can result if no abnormality is found because the proctoscope does not extend vision beyond the first 10 cm of the rectum, and higher lesions may be discounted. A note of the vascular pattern and whether there is bleeding on examination, granularity or ulceration are important features to be recorded. With appropriate training and equipment therapeutic procedures, such as the injection or banding of internal haemorrhoids, can be performed in the surgery.

Equipment and the procedure

A pre-warmed instrument is gradually introduced into the anus with the patient in the left lateral position. A rotatory movement during insertion eases the passage of the instrument and the handle should rest posteriorly. The obdurator is then withdrawn and inspection made.

With most instruments the light source is a battery-powered bulb at the base of the instrument, but an instrument with fibre-optic illumination along its anterior edge gives much better views. Prices of complete instruments vary from £80 to £400, depending largely on the light source. The instruments are available in a variety of diameters and lengths and one with a diameter of approximately 20 mm and a length of approximately 60 mm or more is ideal for use in general practice. Recommended sterilization procedures should be followed.

Sigmoidoscopy

Sigmoidoscopy is an essential part of colonic examination and particularly necessary prior to a barium enema. This is because a barium enema may miss lesions up to the sigmoid and also because an obstructing lesion may prevent the introduction of barium. The instrument also allows biopsies to be taken.

About half of all large bowel cancers may be seen with a rigid sigmoidoscope. Polyps and villous adenomas can also be detected and evidence of bleeding from higher up the gastrointestinal tract may be an indication of significant disease.

The equipment and the procedure

The examination is within the range of the general practitioner. The instrument is usually either 25 or 30 cm in length and either 15 or 20 mm in diameter. Some sigmoidoscopes have a hinged viewing window with a screw tightener, whilst others have a lighting chamber that fits on to the end of the instrument.

Before examination it is important to explain the procedure to the patient. Good patient positioning is critical for a successful examination. The patient either lies in the left lateral or knees to chest position. If in the left lateral position the buttocks need to be positioned at the edge of the bed, with the knees slightly extended. A warmed and lubricated instrument is introduced with a rotatory movement and the obdurator removed after advancing the instrument about 5 cm in the direction of the umbilicus. Thereafter, under direct vision the instrument is advanced in a backward direction along the curve of the sacrum. Air insufflation can be used to push back the mucosa, but this should be kept to a minimum to avoid discomfort. The rectosigmoid junction (10–15 cm) can be difficult to negotiate without patient discomfort and instrumentation is usually limited to around 20 cm. Biopsies may be taken whilst the instrument is slowly withdrawn, utilizing specially designed basket-shaped forceps.

Serious bleeding or perforation are potential complications of sigmoidoscopy and the examination needs to be conducted with care. Fortunately these complications are rare and need not prevent the general practitioner from acquiring the technique.

Flexible sigmoidoscopy

The procedure

Flexible sigmoidoscopy involves the passage of a fibre-optic endoscope into the distal large bowel with the patient in the left lateral position. Examination of the rectum, sigmoid colon, and descending colon up to the splenic flexure or a distance of 60 cm is achieved. The test is easily performed after minimal preparation, such as two disposable phosphate enemas given 30 minutes apart. Sedation is not usually required and the procedure is well tolerated by the patient. In most cases the examination can be carried out in less than 10 minutes.

Indications

The primary indication for flexible sigmoidoscopy is the investigation of rectal bleeding or altered bowel habit. Fibre-optic examination of the sigmoid colon should be carried out in all cases where there is significant diverticulosis, because barium enema examination will easily miss polyps or even carcinoma in the presence of severe diverticular disease. Open-access flexible sigmoidoscopy is now available in several hospitals, but has not yet gained the widespread support which gastroenterologists are now giving to open-access gastroscopy.

Colonoscopy

When a more complete examination of the colon is required a full colonoscopy can be carried out using a much longer fibre-optic instrument which allows the operator to visualize the entire colon including the ascending colon and caecum.

The procedure

The patient needs to be specially prepared the day before, by giving a powerful laxative, such as Picolax (Nordic), in order to cleanse the bowel and allow adequate visualization. Full colonoscopy is usually carried out under intravenous sedation, for example with diazepam, although patients often need analgesia in the form of pethidine. These patients require close monitoring, including pulse oximetry; X-ray screening may also be used. Examination commences with the patient in the left lateral position. The colonoscope is advanced until further insertion produces patient discomfort or retrograde movement of the tip of the colonoscope. This usually indicates the formation of a loop which requires reduction before proceeding. The patient may need to be turned or repositioned to achieve this. X-ray screening facilitates the examination by allowing the endoscopist to see precisely what sort of loop has formed. Full colonoscopy may take 20–30 minutes to complete depending on colonic anatomy and the number of biopsies taken.

Indications

Colonoscopy is indicated in patients with suspected large bowel disease when the barium enema is normal. Other indications for colonoscopy include investigation of iron deficiency anaemia and the full evaluation of inflammatory bowel disease where, for instance, the extent of colitis needs to be accurately established. It is also very useful for the investigation of Crohn's disease, where they may be no abnormality on the left side of the colon but significant disease in the transverse or ascending colon, and in obtaining histology for confirmation of ileo-caecal Crohn's disease. Both colonoscopy and flexible sigmoidoscopy have the advantage over barium enema examination of providing access to tissue for histological analysis. In addition to taking biopsies it is also possible to perform one or two therapeutic procedures through the colonoscope, the most common of which is diathermy snare removal of polyps. This usually only adds a few minutes to the procedure and avoids the need for a laparotomy to be performed especially if the polyp is large and adenomatous. It is also possible to coagulate or inject vascular abnormalities which might be causing occult gastrointestinal blood loss. This condition, known as angiodysplasia, can only be diagnosed by colonoscopy and is another reason why colonoscopy is the investigation of choice for examining the large bowel of patients with occult blood loss.

Double contrast barium enema

The procedure

This technique has now superseded the older technique of single contrast barium radiology, the difference being that the radiologist now attempts to provide a very thin coating of barium over the colonic mucosa with instillation of air into the lumen to provide an adequate contrast. This enables the radiologist to distinguish small lesions which would otherwise be lost in a sea of barium. A well-performed double contrast barium enema examination can yield valuable information about mucosal ulceration, neoplasia, and diverticulosis, but will miss small mucosal lesions, such as angiodysplasia. Preparation is the same as for colonoscopy. It has the advantage over colonoscopy of being less invasive with less risk to the patient. It is also unusual for a barium enema examination not to completely visualize the entire colon, although in some circumstances multiple loops of colon overlying each other make interpretation difficult. This is normally overcome by taking abdominal films in different projections. Unlike colonoscopy, of course, there is no facility for biopsy, although there is the therapeutic opportunity of reducing an intestinal intussusception in infants. Barium enema examination has an advantage over colonoscopy in its ability to detect fistula formation in Crohn's disease.

Indications

Double contrast barium enema is indicated for the further investigation of altered bowel habit or rectal bleeding when proctoscopy and sigmoidoscopy have failed to make a diagnosis or failed to demonstrate the extent of colitis. It is the only way of demonstrating the extent of fistulating Crohn's disease or paracolic abscess.

FUNCTIONAL STUDIES

Gastric function tests

These have largely fallen into disuse following the advent of powerful acid-suppressing drugs, such as H_2-receptor antagonists and, latterly, proton pump inhibitors. Acid output can be measured under basal conditions or in response to stimulation, usually by pentagastrin or occasionally by insulin-induced hypoglycaemia. These tests were used as a measure of the completeness of denervation of the stomach following vagotomy, but they are not routinely used now as they rarely affect patient management. The technique involves the patient swallowing a 14 or 16 mm nasogastric tube which is then positioned to lie along the body of the stomach in a position which allows easy aspiration of gastric secretions. Basal acid output is usually measured before giving a stimulant, such as pentagastrin, following which maximum acid output is measured. There are now very few indications for this sort of test apart from for research studies.

Pancreatic exocrine function tests

There are a variety of ways of measuring pancreatic exocrine function. These can be divided into tests which measure pancreatic secretions directly, utilizing a tube within the duodenum, and tubeless tests. The pancreas is stimulated with either a specifically formulated fatty test meal, such as in the Lundh test, or using a pancreatic stimulant, such as pancreozymin-cholecystokinin, which is given as an infusion based on the patient's weight. The pancreatic secretory responses are then measured in terms of their volume and the amount of bicarbonate and enzymes produced, trypsin being the most commonly measured enzyme. Tubeless tests of pancreatic function are less sensitive but more acceptable to the patient. There are several types of tubeless pancreatic function tests, the most common of which are the para-aminobenzoic acid (PABA) test and pancrealauryl test. The PABA test involves the oral administration of 1 g of para-aminobenzoic acid. Pancreatic enzymes split the amino acid from the parent compound and this is released into the duodenum at a rate depending on the amount of chymotrypsin available. It is then absorbed and excreted in the urine where its measurement provides an indirect measure of pancreatic function. The pancrealauryl test works on a similar principle, utilizing a fluorescein dye which is released and excreted in the urine and measured spectrophotometrically. These tests are less accurate than the Lundh test meal but do provide a valuable screening test for patients with suspected pancreatic insufficiency. The main indication for these tests is the further investigation of steatorrhoea when a small bowel biopsy is normal.

Tests of gall-bladder function

A conventional oral cholecystogram requires a functioning gall-bladder in order for the dye to be concentrated within it, and to some extent this test is a measure of gall-bladder function. Failure to opacify the dye usually indicates a pathological gall-bladder. If the dye is concentrated in the gall-bladder, contraction can also be observed following the administration of a fatty meal. Occasionally, a normal ultrasound scan will miss acalculous gall-bladder disease which can then be picked up on oral cholecystogram.

Indications

An oral cholecystogram is an efficient and cost-effective way of diagnosing gallstones, but has to some extent been replaced by ultrasound examination which is also available on an open-access basis in many areas. An oral cholecystogram is essential if oral dissolution therapy for cholesterol gallstones is contemplated, as failure to opacify indicates a non-functioning gall-bladder.

Laproscopy

This technique has been used for many years by gynaecologists to examine the pelvic viscera. It is occasionally used by gastroenterologists to perform liver biopsy under direct vision for a specific lesion identified on the liver surface. It is not, however, a widely used examination in gastroenterology.

COST IMPLICATIONS OF INVESTIGATIONS

Costs and cost-effectiveness are key words in current medical management. The costs of individual investigations have proved to be difficult to calculate and it is even more daunting to examine the implications of one approach versus another.

In procedure and unit overhead costs the figures shown in Table 2.1 for the Freeman Hospital, Newcastle upon Tyne, were used by the British Society of Gastroenterology working party in their report *Provision of gastrointestinal endoscopy and related services for a district general hospital* (1990).

Table 2.1 *Procedures and unit costs for the Freeman Hospital, Newcastle upon Tyne*

Procedure	Cost (£)
Diagnostic upper gastrointestinal endoscopy	65
Therapeutic upper gastrointestinal endoscopy (stenting)	130
Diagnostic colonscopy	110
Therapeutic colonscopy (polypectomy)	170
Diagnostic ERCP	120*
Therapeutic ERCP	365*

* Plus radiology costs.

The costs of gastroscopy are considerably higher (probably doubled) if cytology or biopsy is performed. These costs are by no means standardized and there is a wide variation, in some instances severalfold, in the figures quoted by different hospitals. The cost of a barium meal examination varies equally and is probably comparable to that of a gastroscopy.

Investigation or a trial of treatment?

A central question with regard to costs is whether a patient with upper gastrointestinal symptoms can be treated without a prior investigation. If it is accepted that patients in certain circumstances can be treated without investigations, then the costs of drug therapy can be balanced against the costs of the potential investigation. At current prices the cost of a four-week course of an ulcer healing drug is approximately half that of a gastroscopy. In some instances patients are subjected to a barium meal followed by a gastroscopy if the results are equivocal, and if biopsies are also taken the total investigation costs are multiplied several times over. At the same time the long-term costs to the health service as well as the community of a missed serious lesion need to be considered.

Consultant referral versus open-access

In addition to the costs of investigation, the implications of referral to hospital need to be taken into account if open-access facilities are not available. Formal referral to hospital leads to an increase in costs in at least two ways: first the costs of intercurrent treatment, and secondly the costs of the out-patient consultations, prior to and after the investigation.

Costs to the patient

These costs, frequently overlooked in assessments of differing management regimes, are compounded by the amount of time taken to obtain relief of symptoms, and by the delays and complications caused by management errors. Measurable factors include the costs of time lost from work, travel, and hospital attendance costs, and an intangible element to cover the 'discomfiture' endured. In considering the overall picture the consequences of management decisions as well as comparative costs need to be considered. A cheaper investigation or drug alternative may be found to be more expensive in the longer term. Simple cost–benefit comparisons do not include intangible costs related to quality of life, and as clinicians our first duty must remain with the patient.

REFERENCES AND FURTHER READING

Bramble, M. G. (1992). Open access endoscopy—a nationwide survey of current practice. *Gut*, **33**, 282–5.

British Society of Gastroenterology (1990). *Provision of gastrointestinal endoscopy and related services for a district general hospital*. British Society of Gastroenterology, London.

Colin-Jones, D. G. (1986). Endoscopy or radiology for upper gastrointestinal symptoms. *Lancet*, **1**, 1022–3.

Cox, T. (1991). Flexible sigmoidoscopy in practice. In *Members handbook 1991*, pp. 345–7. Royal College of General Practitioners, London.

Douglass, R. A. and Hungin, A. S. (1988) Discrepancies in the availability of open access services comparison between the Northern and Oxford regions. *Journal of the Royal College of General Practitioners*, **38**, 28–9.

Hungin, A. S. (1987). Use of an open access gastroscopy service by a general practice. Findings and subsequent referral rate. *Journal of the Royal College of General Practitioners*, **37**, 170–1.

Johnsen, R., Bernersen, B., Straume, B., Forde, O. H., Bostad, L., Burhol, P. G. (1991). Prevalences of endoscopic and histological findings in subjects with and without dyspepsia. *British Medical Journal*, **302**, 749–52.

Jones, R. (1985). Open access endoscopy. *British Medical Journal*, **291**, 424–6.

Kalra, L., Price, W. R., Jones, B. M. J. and Hamlyn, A. N. (1988). Open access fibresigmoidoscopy: a comparative audit of efficacy. *British Medical Journal*, **296**, 1095–6.

Tate, J. J. T. and Royle, G. T. (1988). Open access colonoscopy for suspected colonic neoplasia. *Gut*, **29**, 1322–5.

3 Evaluating upper abdominal pain

Roger Jones

Patients with upper abdominal symptoms account for 3–4 per cent of consultations in general practice, and many of these complain of abdominal pain. The majority will have recurrent, mild to moderate symptoms, with only a small proportion presenting as acute abdominal emergencies. The management of the acute abdomen is well-described in other texts, and is not considered further here. This chapter discusses the evaluation of patients presenting with recurrent upper abdominal discomfort and pain, with particular reference to the selection of patients for investigation, the choice of investigations available, general practitioners' access to these investigations, and the longer-term management of patients with recurrent abdominal pain.

UPPER ABDOMINAL SYMPTOMS

Most upper abdominal symptoms presented to general practitioners are broadly covered by the term dyspepsia, which has been defined in a number of studies as 'upper abdominal or retrosternal pain or discomfort referrable to the upper gastrointestinal tract'. As previously discussed, dyspepsia does not represent a single symptom, but denotes a symptom-complex, in which other complaints, including abdominal discomfort, fullness, belching, flatulence, heartburn, regurgitation, changes in appetite, nausea, and vomiting may all be present to a greater or lesser extent. The 'pathological' correlates of these symptoms include not only gastric and duodenal ulcer, gastric and oesophageal cancer, oesophagitis, and non-ulcer dyspepsia, but also gall-bladder and biliary disease, irritable bowel syndrome, and other causes of abdominal pain, including conditions such as pancreatic cancer and Crohn's disease. The possibility that a group of symptoms could, on the one hand, represent a trivial condition and, on the other hand, a life-threatening one encapsulates the challenge of making appropriate management decisions in patients with upper abdominal pain.

EPIDEMIOLOGY

The early studies of the epidemiology of dyspepsia and peptic ulcer disease in the 1950s and 1960s have already been described. The first studies from general practice in which endoscopy and radiology were used to determine the underlying causes of dyspepsia were published 1970s, and initially reported on 50 consecutive patients with dyspepsia presenting to their general practitioners over a six-month period; specific lesions were discovered in 60 per cent of these. Taking these findings was those of previous studies and extrapolating from them, it was suggested that in a population of 300 000 people served by a single district general hospital there may be as may as 4500 'severe dyspeptics' of whom 60 per cent (2700) have a specific lesion of the upper gastrointestinal tract. In 1982, further studies from Gloucester were published, in which a larger number of patients were examined, and concluded that the prevalence of dyspepsia in the urban practices in Gloucester was 10.4 per 1000 patients, and that in rural practice 10 miles outside the city the prevalence was 27.3 per 1000.

Although these were the first figures obtained from practice-based surveys, they did not permit definite conclusions to be drawn about the natural history of dyspepsia and its relationship to peptic ulceration. There were, however, suggestions from radiological and endoscopic follow-up studies that barium-negative and endoscopy-negative dyspepsia has a favourable outlook in terms of not developing peptic ulceration. Studies from Scandinavia, where 'gastritis' is a very common diagnosis in primary care, had shown that 30–40 per cent of patients with investigation-negative dyspepsia developed ulcers, but these reports were confined to patients attending hospital clinics and relied on radiological assessments. In 1985, an account of the epidemiology of dyspepsia in Göteborg, Sweden was published. This survey reported a peak prevalence (the observation period was unstated) of 26 per cent for dyspepsia in men aged 50 years, making it the fourth most frequent of a list of 30 common symptoms enquired after in a questionnaire study. The prevalence fell to 12 per cent in men aged over 60 years. Similar figures for the prevalence of dyspepsia in women were reported; these results were contrasted with those obtained in a similar study in Denmark, which gave an overall prevalence figure (the observation period was again unstated) for dyspepsia of 27 per cent of the population aged between 15 and 70 years.

In a very large survey from Tromsö in Norway, more than 14 000 middle-aged men and women born between 1925 and 1959 were studied and questioned about, amongst other things, peptic ulcer diagnosis and upper abdominal pain. Peptic ulcers were reported in 5.3 per cent of the men and 2.1 per cent of the women in the study, whilst heartburn and abdominal pain were reported by 16.2 per cent and 12.6 per cent, respectively, of men and 10.1 per cent and 12.3 per cent of women, with symptom prevalence increasing with age over the age range 20–54 years.

The most recent survey of the prevalence of upper abdominal symptoms, performed in Southampton, Birmingham, Nottingham, Glasgow, and Aberdeen has been described in the previous chapter, and found a six-month period prevalence of dyspeptic symptoms in the general population of 38 per cent. In this study symptom frequency fell with increasing age, more markedly in men than in women, whilst consultation rates with general practitioners rose with age. There was a striking degree of overlap between symptoms of upper abdominal pain and heartburn and, in later studies, similar overlap between these symptoms and those of irritable bowel syndrome has also been described. In interview studies with patients identified in community surveys, the presence of a variety of other abdominal symptoms besides dyspepsia was observed. More than half of all the dyspeptic patients also had nausea, heartburn, regurgitation, and abdominal bloating, and reported that their symptoms were made worse by changes in posture.

The natural history of dyspepsia is less well documented. The annual incidence of new cases of dyspepsia has been estimated to be as low as 1.6 per cent, but a group from the Mayo clinic have published a much higher figure of 7.7 per cent in a recent survey. In a study of over 2000 patients identified in a community survey in Hampshire and followed for two years, a 'new dyspepsia' incidence rate of 10–11 per cent per annum was found, with a similar proportion of patients becoming symptom-free each year. In the same period the annual incidence of peptic ulcer disease was about 0.5 per cent. These figures mean that fewer than 1 in 10 patients presenting to general practitioners with dyspeptic symptoms will have a peptic ulcer as a cause for their symptoms, with the majority having a variety of less severe, self-limiting conditions, including non-ulcer dyspepsia, acute gastritis, and minor degrees of gastro-oesophageal reflux disease (GORD).

INTERPRETATION OF SYMPTOMS

Our textbooks are full of 'classical' descriptions of the clinical picture of peptic ulceration, and at least one Royal Physician has asserted that most cases of dyspepsia can be accurately diagnosed on the basis of the clinical history alone. This is manifestly untrue. A number of studies have shown that the provisional diagnosis made by experienced clinicians on the basis of history alone is more often than not at odds with the 'real' diagnosis at endoscopy. The predictive value of many upper gastrointestinal symptoms is rather poor, although a few features of duodenal ulcer disease, such as night pain and pain relieved by eating food, possess reasonable specificity and sensitivity for an accurate final diagnosis. In reflux symptoms, the link between clinical presentation and findings at endoscopy or pH studies is strongest, so that patients with 'typical' reflux symptoms can generally be managed, at least initially, on the basis of symptoms alone. The severity of reflux symptoms is poorly related to the endoscopic and histological severity of the oesophagitis.

However, the arguments surrounding the relationship of symptoms to endoscopic findings are bedevilled by a number of other studies which show that macroscopic and histological abnormalities of the upper gastrointestinal tract are very common in asymptomatic subjects. A significant proportion of the general population, without dyspeptic symptoms, have active duodenal ulceration, and if gastric and duodenal biopsies are examined histologically, a much larger number of abnormalities are found. Added to this is the well-documented observation that many ulcers heal spontaneously. In placebo-controlled trials of ulcer-healing agents, the healing rate on placebo is often as high as 30–40% per cent and, in some studies from Switzerland, has been reported as 70 per cent. These observations challenge the concept of a 'normal' upper gastrointestinal tract and the link between presenting symptoms and endoscopic findings often has to be intepreted with caution. Even in studies which purport to identify early gastric cancer in patients presenting with vague dyspeptic symptoms, it is possible that the finding of malignant or pre-malignant changes are coincidental rather than causally related to patients' symptomatology.

WHICH SYMPTOMS MATTER?

Some guidance has emerged from studies from radiology and endoscopy units, in which patients' clinical features have been linked to the findings on investigation. The most significant aspects of the clinical history appear to be the patient's age, gender (with male sex being a strong predictive factor for peptic ulceration), previous history of ulceration, smoking, and moderate to severe pain relieved by antacids or food. Observations of this kind have formed the basis for rough-and-ready clinical scoring systems, but the accumulation of much larger data sets has also permitted the use of computer-aided diagnosis in patients presenting with upper abdominal pain. The best known of these systems is the Glasgow Dyspepsia System (GLADYS), in which the clinical details of several hundred patients investigated in a gastroenterology unit have been stored; the responses to a structured questionnaire can be used to produce a computer-generated hierarchy of diagnoses. The two main problems with computer-aided diagnosis of this kind have been the poor transferability of data from one country to another, suggesting that certain populations may manifest specific clinical features, and also the complexity of the questionnaires which have to be completed to arrive at a list of diagnoses. The systems currently available have not yet been shown to be sufficiently robust or sufficiently compact for routine use, and certainly have not yet found a place in general practice. A condensed version of the GLADYS approach developed by the Italian dyspepsia project incorporates a much shorter questionnaire, and is said to possess comparable sensitivity and specificity, although once again its evaluation in the primary care setting is still awaited.

A further complicating issue in symptom interpretation is the observation, discussed in an earlier chapter, that the severity and frequency of symptoms and their effect on patients' functional states is a poor predictor of patients' tendency to seek medical care. Initial evaluation in general practice has, therefore, to accommodate not only an attempt to arrive at an accurate 'anatomical' diagnosis, but also to discover the patient's real agenda and anxieties about the significance of the symptoms presented in the surgery. The decision to investigate patients turns not only on the features of the clinical history, which may be suggestive of serious disease, but also on individual physician's perceptions of patients' beliefs and concerns.

An example of the importance of addressing these concerns is a study of the consequences of negative endoscopies. In an open-access service, patients referred by general practitioners for endoscopy with provisional diagnoses of upper gastrointestinal lesions and who were found to have normal or near-normal (minimal gastritis) upper gastrointestinal tracts were studied. When consultation and prescribing rates before endoscopy and in a two-year period after endoscopy were analysed, there was a substantial reduction in frequency of consultation and prescription of all drugs, particularly gastrointestinal preparations, suggesting that the negative findings acted as a powerful therapeutic agent in relieving patients' anxieties.

We may not, of course, always need to refer patients for endoscopy. It seems likely that a patient whose history is heard sympathetically and fully and who receives an appropriate physical examination is just as likely to accept reassurance as if the same conclusion was reached by endoscopy. We should not underestimate the significance for our patients of the consultation and the physical examination.

THE DECISION TO INVESTIGATE

The extent of variation amongst general practitioners in their decisions to investigate patients with upper abdominal symptoms, and some possible reasons for them have been discussed in the previous chapter. There are, however, a number of guide-lines which can be used to inform the decision about whether or not to investigate at an early stage or to defer investigation and treat on the basis of symptoms alone. These guidelines for upper gastrointestinal investigation have recently been published by the British Society of Gastroenterology in a handbook on the provision of endoscopic facilities in District General Hospitals, and are listed below.

1. Think about early investigation.
   (a) Age over 45 years with new dyspepsia.
   (b) Symptoms recur after adequate therapy.
   (c) Recurrent symptoms from a known gastric ulcer.
   (d) Presence of one or more warning features: dysphagia, vomiting, weight loss, bleeding, anaemia.

2. Think twice before investigating.
   (a) Age less than 45 years.
   (b) Known duodenal ulcer.
   (c) No trial of antacids.
   (d) No trial of H_2 blocker.
   (e) Typical reflux symptoms.
   (f) Symptoms suggest irritable bowel syndrome.

Age is a most important factor; this recommendation is based on a number of studies which have shown that the incidence of malignant lesions in patients under the age of 45 years is extremely low. In a large series of endoscopy and radiology examinations from Leicester, for example, all the patients in whom malignant disease was identified were over the age of 45 years. In the same report, a retrospective study of several thousand endoscopies, in which more than 700 patients were found to have upper gastrointestinal malignancy, was analysed; only 1.6 per cent of patients with malignant diseases were under the age of 45 years and all of these were said to have presented with symptoms suggestive of a cause more serious than 'simple dyspepsia'. In the context of downward pressure on that use of investigations, these guidelines are useful in selecting patients who can be regarded as being at 'low' or 'high' risk of serious disease— peptic ulceration or malignancy—permitting the use of time and symptomatic or ulcer-healing therapy as the initial management strategy for patients not falling into the high risk group.

CONFLICTING STRATEGIES

A significant change in thinking is now taking place. Clearly, if malignant disease of the stomach and oesophagus did not exist, many of the arguments about the choice of patients and timing of investigations in upper abdominal symptoms would not be relevant. However, there is continuing anxiety about 'missing' gastric cancer, and the identification of malignant lesions is an important component of the decision about whether or not to investigate. A nihilistic view is, of course, that by the time gastric or oesophageal cancer is diagnosed on the basis of symptoms, the outlook is so awful that it might have been kinder not to have made an early diagnosis at all.

More recent work, aimed at earlier detection of gastric cancer, casts doubts on these rather traditional views. In a study from Birmingham, for example, in which dyspeptic patients are admitted to a 'fast track' dyspepsia investigation service, Fielding's group have claimed that more than 10 per cent of patients can be shown, when endoscopic biopsies are carefully examined, to have dysplastic or metaplastic changes in the gastric mucosa which may well be pre-malignant and are thought to require endoscopic surveillance. If this is true, and early endoscopy represents an important strategy for early diagnosis of gastric cancer, then we have to re-think some of our preconceptions about immediate and deferred investigation. In the early days of open-access endoscopy, better access for general practitioners to endoscopy did not seem to be associated with earlier diagnosis of gastric cancer or a better prognosis for the disease. The final evidence in this debate is not yet available, but is awaited with considerable interest.

Of more obvious significance is a consideration of the costs involved in adopting either an early endoscopy strategy or an expectant approach, involving symptomatic treatment and endoscopy only if symptoms persist or recur. Two important studies have cast doubt on the view that delaying endoscopy, even in a low risk patients, is associated with cost savings. A research group from New South Wales have compared the two strategies; in Australia it is not possible to obtain reimbursement for the cost of H_2-receptor antagonists unless a definite endoscopic or radiological diagnosis of peptic ulceration or ulcerative oesophagitis has been made. In this study 139 patients were randomized to 'Australian' management, in which ulcer-healing drugs were given only after a positive investigation or to a 'British' group, in which general practitioners were able to treat freely, without the need for investigation, although in both groups the option to investigate or refer was always open. Patients were followed for six months and the costs associated with each strategy were carefully calculated, and included not only direct costs in primary and secondary health care, but also prescribing costs and costs to the patient and the social security services. The cumulative investigation rate in the 'Australian' group was approximately 75 per cent at six months, with the rate for the 'British' group being less than half this. Most significantly, the final costs of investigation and treatment in each group were almost identical, around 400 Australian dollars, and there were no significant differences in clinical outcome in either group.

A study from Sweden has recently compared three strategies:

1. Initial H_2-receptor antagonist treatment to all patients, followed by endoscopy if therapy failed to alleviate the symptoms or if symptoms recurred.
2. Initial symptomatic treatment with antacids to all patients, followed by

endoscopy in those still symtomatic after 2–4 weeks and H_2-receptor antagonist treatment only in those with acid-related diseases (peptic ulcer, duodenitis, and oesophagitis).
3. Initial endoscopy in all patients, with H_2-recepter antagonist treatment being given only to those with acid-related diseases.

This was a theoretical analysis, the observation period was one year after initial consultation and in Sweden 65 000 individuals would have been expected to make 104 600 consultations in the study period. The authors assumed that 20 per cent would have 'casual' symptoms which would be self-limiting and would resolve in two weeks with or without treatment, and that 30 per cent would have acid-related diseases. The accuracy of these figures is open to question, but they may well represent clinical experience in Sweden. A further assumption was that 65 per cent of the patients in strategy (1) would undergo endoscopy due to failure of treatment or recurrence of symptoms. Finally, the authors postulated that an endoscopic diagnosis would rationalize treatment in organic dyspepsia and elevate anxiety in functional dyspepsia, so that subsequent consultations were reduced by 50 per cent. These seem reasonable assumptions, based on some of the studies mentioned earlier. The costs of consultation, endoscopy and H_2-receptor treatment were included in the analysis and H_2-blocker therapy was assumed to reduce absenteeism from work by 40 per cent, whilst the reassurance of a negative endoscopy was thought to reduce absenteeism in 'functional' dyspepsia by only 5 per cent. This may also be an under-estimate.

The conclusions of this study were that the total costs varied surprisingly little between the three strategies; the total cost, in 1991 figures and US dollars for the population under study was predicted to be approximately $83 million for strategy (1), $82 million for strategy (2), and $76 million for strategy (3). In other words, the initial endoscopy strategy appeared to have a slight advantage in terms of resource utilization.

These studies have to be taken seriously, particularly when other authors have suggested that even if endoscopy is initially deferred, between 60 and 70 per cent of all dyspeptic patients will end up having an investigation at some stage. In the epidemiological surveys undertaken in Southampton, the percentage of the general population who had been investigated with either a barium meal or an endoscopy was of the order of 20 per cent, emphasizing the lifetime frequency of investigations for upper abdominal complaints.

It may well be, therefore, that even in a time of shrinking resources, early endoscopy followed by rational therapy offers not only the most cost-effective approach to the management of patients with upper abdominal symptoms, but may also be associated with the earlier diagnosis of gastric and oesophageal cancer. The results of clinical studies on early endoscopy and early gastric cancer are now eagerly anticipated, and it would be appropriate for a prospective trial along the lines of the work by Goulston and Lindberg to be undertaken in this country.

COSTS OF DYSPEPSIA

An account of the modern treatment of gastric and duodenal ulcer disease is provided in a later chapter, but the evaluation and treatment of non-ulcer dyspepsia remains controversial and a variety of management options are available. It is important to recognize that, as well as carrying significant prescribing costs, functional dyspepsia itself has considerable economic consequences. The only published cost analysis of functional dyspepsia once again comes from Sweden, and appeared more than ten years ago. The estimated annual cost was 457 million US dollars, (944 million US dollars in 1991 prices), or 113 630 US dollars per 1000 population per year. These estimates did not include the costs of investigations, and recent changes in prescribing habits may have further increased the contribution of drug costs. All of these costs are, however, overshadowed by costs for absenteeism, which have proved to be unexpectedly large when ascertained objectively. The situation in Sweden, where there is a social insurance scheme with high accessibility and generous terms for compensation, may be atypical, but it is important to recognize that adequate treatment of upper abdominal symptoms is important in a socio-economic, as well as a clinical, context.

TREATMENT OF NON-ULCER DYSPEPSIA

Initial trials of acid-suppressing therapy in patients with non-ulcer dyspepsia were disappointing. This negative therapeutic effect could have been predicted, because at the time that most of these trials were undertaken, sub-division of dyspepsia into ulcer-like, reflux-like, dysmotility-like, and idiopathic dyspepsia was unusual, and patients with negative investigations tended to be grouped together. Acid-suppressing therapy would have been inappropriate for a substantial proportion of these patients with other causes for their symptoms, almost certainly explaining the negative results of many trials of H_2-recepter antagonists in non-ulcer dyspepsia.

However, the report of the international working party, recommending the classification of dyspepsia into different types has helped in terms of clinical management, and has also heightened research awareness of the need to classify patients accurately before entering them into therapeutic trials. A further development of this approach has been the innovative use of single-subject studies conducted in Trondheim, Norway. Recognizing that in many functional gastrointestinal disorders therapeutic responses may be idiosyncratic and not always easy to predict on clinical symptoms, the single-subject trial has been developed to permit short courses of therapy, lasting for as little as one day, to be randomly alternated with placebo while subjects keep a diary record of symptoms each day. Using this technique it is possible to determine quite quickly the extent of therapeutic response to, for example, an H_2-receptor antagonist, although there is no reason why this approach could not be used to investigate the effects of other drugs used in the treatment of non-ulcer dyspepsia. Following the international working party's classification, acid-suppressing agents can be thought of as appropriate treatment for ulcer-like dyspepsia and for some patients with reflux-like dyspepsia, although others in this group may benefit from taking agents aimed at changing oesophago-gastric motility and improving lower oesophageal sphincter function. Patients with characteristics of dysmotility-like dyspepsia are much less likely to benefit from this treatment, and an approach based on explanation and dietary modification, backed up by the use of bulking agents, anti-diarrhoeals, and anti-spasmodics if appropriate, is more likely to succeed.

It is also worth emphasizing the importance of thinking about the influence of life-style on digestive symptoms. Just as smoking and alcohol, for example, are risk factors for inflammatory and neoplastic change in the upper gastrointestinal tract, so they may be associated with dyspeptic and reflux symptoms. Rapid eating and air swallowing, sometimes in association with anxiety, may also lead to upper gastrointestinal symptoms as well as abdominal bloating. Provocation of symptoms by specific foodstuffs, by eating too quickly, and by tension and anxiety, also need to be considered as remediably causes for non-ulcer dyspepsia. Patients' undeclared concern about the possibility that their symptoms represent a serious or potentially fatal illness may, on occasion, overshadow the influence of these other factors.

FURTHER READING

British Society of Gastroenterology (1990). *Provision of gastrointestinal endoscopy and related services for a district general hospital.* British Society of Gastro-enterology, London.

Capurso, L., Koch, M. M., Dezi, A., DiCiocco, U. and the Gruppo Operativo Dispepsia (1988). Towards a quantitative diagnosis of dyspepsia: the value of clinical symptoms. *Italian Journal of Gastroenterology*, **20**, 191–202.

Colin-Jones, D. G. (1988). Management of dyspepsia: report of a working party. *Lancet*, **1**, 576–9.

Gear, M. W. L., Ormiston, M. C., Barnes, R. J., Rocyn-Jones, J. and Voss, G. C. (1980). Endoscopic studies of dyspepsia in the community: an 'open access', service. *British Medical Journal*, **280**, 1135–7.

Goulston, K. H., Dent, O. F., Mant, A., Logan, J., Nau, M. (1991). Use of H_2-receptor antagonists in patients with dyspepsia and heartburn: a cost comparison. *Medical Journal of Australia*, **155**, 20–6.

Hallissey, M. T., Allum, W. H., Jewkes, A. J., Ellis, D. J., and Fielding, J. W. L. (1990). Early detection of gastric cancer. *British Medical Journal*, **301**, 513–15.

Holdstock, G., Harman, M., Machin, D., Patel, C. and Lloyd, R. S. (1986). Prospective testing of a scoring system designed to improve case selection for upper gastrointestinal investigation. *Gastroenterology*, **90**, 1164–9.

Johannessen, T. (1991). Controlled trials in single subjects. *British Medical Journal*, **303**, 173–4.

Jones, R. (1988). What happens to patients with non-ulcer dyspepsia after endoscopy? *Practitioner*, **232**, 75–8.

Knill Jones, R. P., Dunwoodie, W. M., and Crean, G. P. (1985). A computer-assisted diagnostic decision system for dyspepsia. In *Decision making in general practice*, eds M. Sheldon, J. Brooke and A. Rector. Macmillan, London.

Nyren, O., Adami, H.-O., Bates, S., Bergstrom, R., and Gustavsson, S. (1986). Absence of therapeutic benefit from antacids or cimetidine for non-ulcer dyspepsia. *New England Journal of Medicine*, **314**, 339–43.

Nyren, O., Lindberg, G., Lindström, E., Marke, L.-A., and Seensalu, R. (1992). Economic costs of functional dyspepsia. *PharmacoEconomics*, **1** (5), 312–24.

Williams, B., Luckas, M., Ellingham, J. H. M., Dain, A., Wicks, A. C. B., Loof, L. and Nyberg, A. (1988). Do young patients with dyspepsia need investigation? *Lancet*, **2**, 1349–51.

4 Gastrointestinal problems in children

Toni Rolles and Christopher Rolles

Gastrointestinal symptoms are a common reason for parents to bring their children to general practitioners and for general practitioners to refer children to hospital. The symptoms may be very obvious or embarrassing and they may be particularly worrying to parents because they are often concerned with activities which have special associations for parenting in the early years of life, such as feeding and potty training, by which the parents judge themselves and feel that they are being judged by other people. This chapter is written by a general practitioner and a hospital paediatrician, who are married to each other and have four children. It offers a practical guide for general practitioners and, perhaps more importantly, an approach which is a synthesis of the authors' experience, both as doctors and parents.

GASTROINTESTINAL DISEASE IN CHILDREN

The pattern of gastrointestinal disease in children is different from that found in adults. In adults, gastrointestinal symptoms usually represent trouble within the gastrointestinal tract, but in children this is often not the case. For example, in children, both vomiting and diarrhoea can be caused by urinary tract infection or otitis media. Adults presenting to a general practitioner with gastrointestinal symptoms are often found to have specific pathology—diverticulitis, peptic ulceration, neoplasia, or cholelithiasis. Minor symptoms and infections are usually treated at home. Conversely, children presenting with gastrointestinal symptoms usually have transient and self-limiting conditions which cannot be labelled specifically, but even these minor symptoms may cause disproportionate anxiety to the parents, and sometimes to the general practitioner, because of poor localization.

An essential part of good practice is understanding the diagnostic probabilities in any given clinical context. The diagnostic probabilities of some childhood gastrointestinal symptoms within general practice are outlined in Table 4.1. So, for example, when presented with a three-year-old with recent onset of loose stools, it would be inappropriate to assume cow's milk allergy and immediately start an exclusion diet, disrupting

Table 4.1 *Diagnostic probabilities of some gastrointestinal presentations in a general paediatric context*

Problem	Possible diagnoses		
	Likely	Fairly unlikely	Very unlikely

Recurrent dull abdominal pain in toddler or older child	No organic cause
	    Constipation
	        Abdominal migraine
	            Pyelonephritis
	                Sexual abuse
	                    Peptic ulceration
	                        Lead poisoning
	                            Porphyria		

Intermittent vomiting in a baby	Physiological possetter
	    Gastro-oesophogeal reflux
	        Urinary tract infection
	            Early or atypical pyloric stenosis
	                Hiatus hernia
	                    Malrotation of gut		

Constipated baby, occasional blood in stools	Physiological variation
	    Dietary factors
	        Breast-feeding
		Cow's milk allergy
		Hirschsprung's
		Hypothyroidism	

Persistent loose stools in toddler or older child	Toddler diarrhoea
	    High laxative diet
	        Persistent bacterial or protozoal infection
	            Lactase deficiency following acute gastro-
	                enteritis
	                Cow's milk protein allergy
	                    Intermittent volvulus
	                        Carcinoid
	                            Inflammatory bowel disease		

Jaundiced neonate	Physiological
	    Breast-milk jaundice
	        Umbilical, urinary tract infection
	            Congenital infection
	                Hypothyroidism
	                    Biliary atresia
	                        Neonatal hepatitis
	                            Galactosaemia
	                                Cystic fibrosis		

family life and assigning a sickness label. However, a good general practitioner should be aware of the signs suggesting more serious disease and would, for example, recognize that a child with weight loss, smelly pale stools, and a pot belly, probably justifies early referral.

In all paediatric consultations the history is given, or at least strongly influenced, by a third party (and sometimes even fourth, fifth, and sixth parties). Remember that it is overlaid with parental perceptions, interpretations, and anxieties. Listen carefully to what the parent has to say, at the same time watching the child. Common sense sometimes indicates that there is a mismatch between what the parent has to say and what you observe. For example, a mother may tell you that her child has been vomiting every feed for the past two days and has copious diarrhoea. Meanwhile the child sits on her lap pink, cheerful, well hydrated, laughing at you. Alternatively, parents may play down their child's problems if, for whatever reason, they feel self-conscious or guilty about bringing the child to the doctor. A careful examination of the child may be helpful and very reassuring, both to oneself and to the parents. However, if the child is very distressed an attempted examination may be unjustified and futile and add very little to what has already been gathered from the history and simple observation. When considering a gastrointestinal problem it may be far more relevant to examine the stool or to observe the pattern of vomiting or feeding than to hold down a screaming child while palpating his or her rigid abdomen. Two essential tools in paediatric gastroenterology are, first, simple diaries relating symptoms to life events and diet and, secondly, weight charts, which show everyone concerned the pattern of a child's growth and how it relates to the norm. There may be situations in which you feel the parents' anxieties are disproportionate. Take time to explore whether these anxieties actually relate to the presenting symptoms or whether they represent entirely different problems.

THE CHILD WHO IS VOMITING

Recurrent vomiting

Children often vomit. They 'mewl and puke'. Vomiting and diarrhoea, like coughing, may be regarded as natural defences for rejecting noxious substances. The cardiac sphincter is relatively underdeveloped in the younger child and this adds to the ease of vomiting. So, the effortless regurgitation or possetting of small quantities of food immediately after feeds, or even for up to one hour or so after lying down, by an otherwise well child who is gaining weight, can be quite normal. Regurgitation of larger volumes, which are occasionally blood-stained, may indicate reflux beyond the normal range or even a hiatus hernia, although this is quite uncommon.

All but the most serious of these conditions will resolve as the baby grows and becomes more upright. Previously, many of these children were referred to hospital, investigated extensively, and often treated surgically. The modern approach is to observe and treat symptomatically; very few will need surgery. However, it is easy to understand that a persistently vomiting child, even when apparently otherwise well, can be a source of great anxiety to the parents. A sensible general practice approach is to take a careful history, to try to observe the child feeding or to get the health visitor to do so, and to examine the child carefully. Weigh the child naked. If you are happy with his or her general condition explain the situation to the parents and suggest that the child is fed sitting up and kept in an upright position for half an hour or so after feeds. Regurgitation can be further reduced by using infant Gaviscon or thickening the feed with a proprietary thickener, such as Carobel or Nestargel, or by increasing the solid component of the feed if the child is weaned. Arrange to see the child again, perhaps in one week, to discuss progress and again weigh the child naked. If the parents see that the child is gaining weight and you have given them a realistic expectation of the natural history of the condition, they will probably be quite happy to accept this management, which could be carried on by the health visitor. However, if at any time there is evidence the child is failing to thrive, you should refer on immediately. The hospital paediatrician has the advantage that he or she can admit the child for observation and parental instruction, although in the long run his or her approach may be the same as yours.

Even in an older child who is otherwise well, recurrent vomiting without other symptoms is unlikely to represent significant organic pathology, although it may be an indicator of emotional or social problems. Check the urine and weigh the child. Asking the parents or an older child him or herself to keep a diary of symptoms can be very useful. It may put the symptoms in perspective for the family, allowing them to see their true frequency. It may actually pin-point certain trigger factors. Together with weighing, it will form part of an ongoing review which can allow the doctor to use time to see if other physical or emotional problems will declare themselves.

Acute vomiting

We have discussed a conservative approach towards recurrent vomiting in an otherwise well child. The sudden onset of vomiting in a previously well child who is now clearly unwell has a very different significance and demands a very different response from the doctor. Faced with a child with acute onset of vomiting, who is clearly unwell and who may or may not have associated symptoms, such as diarrhoea, evidence of abdominal pain, or fever, the general practitioner has to answer the following questions.

1. *Is this gastroenteritis?* Gastroenteritis is usually characterized by both vomiting and diarrhoea but, on occasions, either symptom may predominate or exist alone. Vomiting will occur during or immediately after a feed and the stomach is obviously trying to empty itself completely. Diarrhoea may follow the onset of vomiting by several hours or even days. Occasionally, a child has occult diarrhoea in which the liquid stools have not been passed but accumulate in the colon causing distension and discomfort. The stool may simply be loose or very watery and occasionally, blood-stained with mucus.

2. *Do these symptoms represent an infection outside the gastrointestinal tract?* We have already said that children often vomit. They vomit readily with generalized infections—septicaemia and some viral illnesses—with infections of the upper and lower respiratory tracts, and particularly of the urinary tract where the vomiting may be very forceful. An older child may give clues localizing the infection to the urinary tract, but a baby or small child hardly ever does. It is vital to consider the possibility of urinary tract infection in a febrile vomiting child with no localizing signs, since the sequelae of missed urinary tract infection can be disastrous. Infection within the central nervous system often causes vomiting, but this will usually be one of a collection of symptoms— extreme irritability or profound apathy, altered level of consciousness, convulsion, neck stiffness—which point one in the right direction. Vomiting may also be a feature of the prodrome of infective hepatitis when it is often associated with upper abdominal tenderness.

3. *Do these symptoms represent a surgical condition somewhere in the gastrointestinal tract?* Forceful vomiting coming on immediately the child starts feeding after birth or early in the neonatal period must suggest intestinal obstruction due to some congenital abnormality until proved otherwise. This is extremely rare but may come the way of general practitioners involved with maternity units and is an indication for immediate referral.

Pyloric stenosis is more common and an average general practitioner will see a case every few years. Typically, the baby is about six weeks old, often male, first-born, is feeding ravenously, may be constipated, and is losing weight. The parents give a typical history of projectile vomiting immediately after feeds. 'Projectile' indicates that the vomit squirts out, landing several feet away from the child. At first the vomiting may be intermittent but becomes persistent. Diagnosis will largely be made on the history but when pyloric stenosis is suspected a feed should be observed. Visible peristalsis may be seen crossing the upper abdomen. Traditionally, a pyloric tumour should be felt, but this can be very difficult unless the observer is experienced and its absence should not negate the diagnosis. Atypical and milder forms may present in a slightly older baby, often a girl, and may be a diagnostic puzzle even to the paediatrician.

Vomiting may also be a feature of intussusception. This occurs mainly in children between the ages of three months and two years and is characterized by the child having spasms of severe abdominal pain. There may be constipation and/or the passage of small quantities of blood-stained mucus rectally. In older children acute vomiting may be a presentation of appendicitis.

4. *Has the child ingested something toxic?* Toddlers and small children are naturally curious about their environment and are likely to eat anything they find, including brightly coloured tablets, medicines, or household fluids in interesting-looking bottles. Many of these substances taste horrible, thus ensuring that not much is swallowed or that reflex protective vomiting occurs immediately. If the ingested substance was caustic or a hydrocarbon, such as paraffin or white spirit, the actual swallowing and the secondary effects of vomiting and possible aspiration into the lungs may be very damaging. A small child can be killed by a very small amount of a toxic substance. Six iron tablets are sufficient to kill a toddler. The diagnosis of toxic ingestion should always be considered in a child who has been quite well up to the time of vomiting. If there is any doubt, the child should be admitted. The appearance and smell of the vomit may be helpful. The general practice approach will depend on the speed with which secondary help is available. There is little point in attempting to empty the stomach after four hours unless the ingested substance was a salicylate or an anticholinergic, such as a tricyclic anti-depressant. If admission is likely to be delayed it may be worthwhile trying to induce vomiting, providing you are absolutely certain that the ingested substance was not caustic or a hydrocarbon. In these cases milk may be helpful in limiting the damage. Vomiting may be induced by mechanical stimulation of the back of the throat, or by giving ipecacuanha paediatric emetic draft (1–2 years 10 ml; over 2 years 15 ml) followed by 300–500 ml of fruit squash or milk and water 50 per cent mixture. The dose can be repeated once after 30 minutes if vomiting has not occurred. Salt water should never be used because of the dangers of salt intoxication in a small child.

5. *Is something else occurring?* Accidental or non-accidental injury, causing fracture, may rarely present as acute vomiting. Space-occupying lesions in the central nervous system may also present as acute, but more usually subacute or chronic, vomiting. As with infections of the central nervous system, there are likely to be other symptoms and signs pointing to the correct localization.

Management of acute vomiting

The management of acute vomiting in childhood is the management of the underlying condition. Each of the many diagnoses which could be made in this situation has its own appropriate management. It is hard to justify the use of anti-emetics in childhood, except as a part of terminal care, and this is particularly true when the doctor is not sure what is occurring and when potentially serious conditions could be masked. The main concern must be to maintain the child's hydration while waiting for the situation to resolve or for the diagnosis to declare itself. It is reasonable in these situations to use oral rehydration fluids, as described below in the section on gastroenteritis.

GASTROENTERITIS

Gastroenteritis implies the inflammation of the whole gut—stomach, small bowel, and colon—but, sometimes symptoms seem to suggest that one area is particularly affected. The inflamed stomach rejects most food and drink, together with acid. More rapid transit through the small bowel results in substantial loss of water and electrolytes, particularly sodium, and of the brush border which temporarily hampers digestion. Rapid transit through the large bowel results in further loss of water. Depending on the severity of the infection, dehydration and loss of electrolytes may be rapid. The smaller the child the greater his or her relative fluid requirements and the more rapid his or her possible dehydration and electrolyte disturbance. In the Third World gastroenteritis is still a major cause of death. In Northern Europe it is usually a fairly benign and self-limiting condition, but it can still be serious, particularly in vulnerable children such as those who are failing to thrive for other reasons.

The inflammation is usually infective but can be due to toxins, for example in staphylococcal food poisoning. The infective organisms vary geographically and with the seasons but are predominantly viral (rotavirus, enterovirus). Less commonly, the infecting organism is bacterial (*Salmonella, Campylobacter, Shigella*, enteropathic *E. coli*) or protozoal (*Giardia, Cryptosporidium*). In the acute stage, the clinical picture may give some clues to the aetiology. For example, blood in the stools is more common with *Campylobacter* and *Shigella. Giardia* presents predominantly as an enteritis without vomiting and with fatty stools. However, finding the infecting organism is largely academic and, unless there are compelling epidemiological or public health reasons, (for example, if the mother is a school cook, there are several children in the same playgroup affected, or the child has just arrived in the UK from India), there are no indications for sending a stool culture for analysis in acute gastroenteritis. Whatever the infecting organism, the initial management is the same. Bacterial gastroenteritis appears to resolve almost as quickly without treatment and there is evidence that treatment with antibiotics prolongs the carrier state and the duration of the diarrhoea. Stool culture will only become necessary in the very few cases where symptoms persist after the acute phase.

Having made a diagnosis of gastroenteritis, the general practitioner must decide how ill the child is and whether he or she can be managed at home. Factors influencing this decision include clinical assessment of the child, knowledge of the parents' capabilities, the home circumstances, how long the child has been ill, whether any treatment is already being given, and whether the doctor will be available to review the child.

Clinically the child is likely to be somewhere between two extremes. At one end of the scale there is a child who is alert with sufficient energy to respond to overtures, either cheerfully or aggressively, who has sufficient muscle tone to sit up on his or her mother's lap or walk into the surgery, whose fontanelle is appropriately full or whose skin turgor is good, whose pulse rate is fairly steady, whose colour is reasonable, and whose nappy is wet or who is passing urine almost normally. At the other end of the scale there is a child who is completely limp and lies across his or her mother's lap and who has only sufficient energy to respond to examination with a whimper. The child is pale, has either a concave fontanelle or has lost skin elasticity. The child's eyes appear sunken. His or her nappy is dry and mother says that he or she has not passed urine for some hours. He or she has a tachycardia and a thin pulse. Weight loss, as an indicator of dehydration in general practice, is not often useful. Previous weights, if available, are likely to have been on different scales in various states of undress, and common sense clinical assessment is usually more relevant. For the purposes of discussion, this clinical assessment scale is represented in Fig. 4.1. Clearly, children in the lower part of the scale, between A and B, should be admitted immediately, but the decision to admit children in other parts of the scale must be based on some of the other factors discussed. So, for example, a confident and experienced doctor who knows that he or she will be available to review the child in a few hours time and who knows that the parents are capable, might decide to keep the child between C and B at home. If, however, the same child had already been given Dioralyte by it's sensible mother for 24 hours and was not responding, the doctor would probably decide to admit. It would be reasonable to keep a child between D and C at home initially, but the doctor might decide to admit if he or she knew that parental anxiety was great and the support network poor.

The aim of management is to maintain hydration and electrolyte balance while the gastrointestinal tract heals itself. In an artificially fed baby, or in children who have been weaned, this is done by stopping all solid food and milk and giving appropriate volumes of appropriate clear fluids. Breast-fed

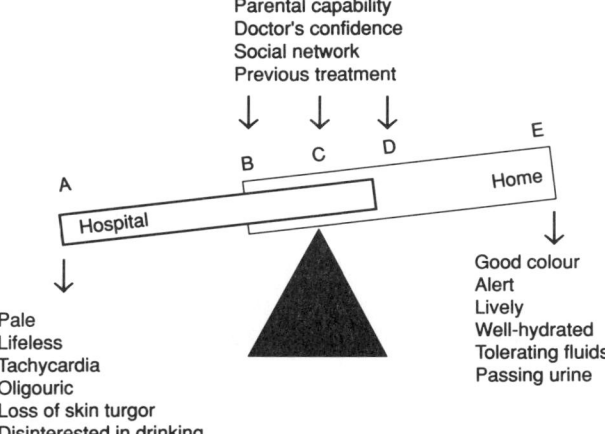

Parental capability
Doctor's confidence
Social network
Previous treatment

B   C   D   E

A   Home

Hospital

Good colour
Alert
Lively
Pale   Well-hydrated
Lifeless   Tolerating fluids
Tachycardia   Passing urine
Oligouric
Loss of skin turgor
Disinterested in drinking

Fig. 4.1 Gastroenteritis clinical assessment scale.

babies should continue at the breast on demand. The breast is unlikely to respond rapidly enough to meet the increased demand for fluid, and so clear fluids should be given in addition to breast milk. The question is, what clear fluid and how much? In all but the very mildest cases, commercial oral rehydration therapy (ORT) probably has advantages over home-made clear fluid, which can be made simply by adding five level teaspoonfuls (25 g) of sugar to a pint (540 ml) of water, producing an approximately isotonic solution. Addition of salt can be very haphazard. In mild cases, it is safer to omit it. Indeed in mild cases the child should be given whatever clear fluid he or she likes best. Ice lollies or ice-cubes are often well tolerated. The commercial ORT solutions, for example Dioralyte, Rehydrat, are relatively cheap and their only danger is if they are made up incorrectly. This may seem self-evident, but it should be stressed that the instructions on the sachets should be followed absolutely, thus producing an isotonic solution which is the basis for their efficacy. Some parents may not be able to read the instructions; others may feel that if the solution is good a stronger solution will be even better; many families will have no way of accurately measuring the volume of liquid required. Bottled water may have extremely variable, often very high, levels of solutes and should not be used to reconstitute ORT. ORT provides a specific balance of sodium and glucose which allows the fluid to be retained in the stomach without being rejected and, once in the small gut, the glucose facilitates the absorption of sodium and water. The fluid should be given in small quantities every few minutes rather than in one large bottle or cupful. How much should be given? Probably much more than you realize. A rough indication of normal fluid requirement according to the

Table 4.2 *Fluid requirement according to body weight*

Body weight (kg)	Normal fluid requirement* (ml/kg/24 h)
< 10	100–120
10–30	60–90
> 30	40–90

* + 5 per cent in mild dehydration, + 10 per cent in moderate dehydration.

child's size is given in Table 4.2. To correct fluid deficit and to allow for continuing excess fluid loss through vomiting and diarrhoea and for lack of parental enthusiasm a volume equal to normal requirement plus 20–30 per cent should be prescribed. If, however, the child still appears thirsty and is willing to take more, there is no danger of over-hydration.

Having started home management it is vital to arrange review. In the mildest cases this may simply consist of telling the parents what to look out for and at what point they should contact you again if things do not proceed according to plan, but, as you proceed down the clinical scale, arrangements should be made for actual review by the doctor. If after a few hours the child is not tolerating properly given oral rehydration fluids and if he or she appears to be moving down the clinical scale, hospital admission should be considered. If the child is tolerating oral rehydration fluids and improving clinically, advice should be given to continue this treatment until the symptoms have settled for some hours. By this time the child will be extremely hungry and most parents will have capitulated and fed him. In the past it was felt necessary after acute gastroenteritis to reintroduce food very gradually, milk feeds being given in increasing strengths over several days. This regrading is now thought to be unnecessary and, once the symptoms have well and truly settled, the child can be started back on his or her normal diet.

There is absolutely no place for the use of anti-diarrhoeals or anti-emetics in acute gastroenteritis, although some parents will have given their children kaolin and morphine, sometimes at the advice of the local pharmacist, by the time they present. Opiates and kaolin may stop or reduce the actual expulsion of diarrhoea, but they do nothing for the loss of fluids and electrolytes through the gut wall, and these accumulate within the gut, giving a false impression of the clinical state and possibly masking weight loss. If the infection is bacterial, slowing the gut down with opiates may actually hinder the expulsion of bacterial toxins and prolong the infection. There is also no place for the use of antibiotics in acute gastroenteritis. The only place in which antibiotics may have a role is when an acute gastroenteritis goes into a chronic state and microbiologically there is a proven residual infection with one or two specific organisms (see below). Remember that in the acute state almost all of the commonly used antibiotics may actually irritate the bowel, thus causing further damage. Antibiotics used casually very frequently prolong the carrier state and induce resistance.

Most children with gastroenteritis can be managed at home. Involvement of the parents will probably allow subsequent episodes to be managed by them alone, without recourse to the doctor.

Problems persisting after acute gastroenteritis

Sometimes a parent will bring a child back to the doctor a few weeks after an episode of acute gastroenteritis complaining that he or she has persistent diarrhoea. Our impression is that this is now occurring less frequently than before. At this point the general practitioner must consider the persistence of a bacterial or protozoal infection and send a stool sample off to the laboratory. The most likely organisms to cause persisting symptoms are *Campylobacter*, *Salmonella*, *Giardia* or *Cryptosporidium*. It is sensible to speak to the microbiologist about requirements for stool culture and also local recommendations for treatment. For example, most laboratories will require at least three stool samples on consecutive days to look for *Giardia* and it probably cannot be ruled out until six samples have been examined. *Giardia* can usually be treated successfully with a 3 day course of metronidazole (7–8 mg per kg body weight three times daily for children between 4 weeks and 12 years of age, adult dose above 12 years of age). It was previously thought to be a rather exotic organism, but modern microbiological techniques are isolating it more frequently, suggesting it may be endemic in parts of the UK. Isolation may still be laborious so, if the clinical picture suggests giardiasis, it would be reasonable to treat empirically. It is debatable whether *Salmonella* and *Campylobacter* need treatment. *Campylobacter* will respond to erythromycin and *Salmonella* to ciprofloxacin, but this is not licensed for children under the age of 8 years at present and the alternatives are much less satisfactory because they may prolong the carrier state. Treatment should be discussed with the microbiologist and the local Public Health laboratory. There is no treatment for *Cryptosporidium*, which can cause large outbreaks of gastroenteritis, but is often carried asymptomatically in stools. It is not killed by chemical treatment of water, but only by sand filtration, which is not carried out routinely in all UK water purification plants. Although it causes a mild disease in most people, it can kill an individual who is immunosuppressed for whatever reason—chemotherapy, high dose steroids or AIDS. The general practitioner should be aware of this and act accordingly. In most cases stool cultures will be negative and the diarrhoea will have settled down within a few weeks. The explanation may be that the acute infection had disorganized the usual colonic flora which, given time, has sorted itself out.

Sometimes the diarrhoea persists and, in these cases, one must consider a persisting lactase deficiency or even a true cow's milk protein allergy which can be triggered by acute gastroenteritis. However, it must be stressed that true cow's milk protein allergy is extremely rare. For example, a project involving four large district general hospitals in the south of England failed to identify a single confirmed case of cow's milk protein allergy in one year. A distinguishing feature between lactose intolerance and cow's milk protein allergy is that lactose intolerance is directly dose-dependent, whereas cow's milk protein allergy is not. So, for example, a child with lactose intolerance may be asymptomatic on half a cup of milk, but increasingly symptomatic as the quantity of milk increases. In contrast, a child with cow's milk protein allergy will be symptomatic on even minute amounts of cow's milk protein. This is understandable when we consider the pathogenesis of lactose intolerance. During acute gastroenteritis, the brush border of the small intestine is swept away, together with the sugar-splitting enzymes lactase, sucrase, and isomaltase. Lactase, being produced at the summit of the villi, is most affected. In most children this is a temporary deficiency, but if it persists, when milk-containing foods are reintroduced, the lactose in the milk acts rather like lactulose, producing diarrhoea. Lactase deficiency is fairly simply diagnosed by finding reducing substances in the stool and Fig. 4.2 shows how this can be done using Clinitest tablets. The stool must be very fresh, so using the hospital laboratory may be impracticable. Diagnosis can also be made by withdrawing all milk-containing products for a few days and then formally challenging the child with lactose, by either fully re-introducing milk-containing products or, as in hospital practice, using powdered lactose in a single dose (2 g per kg both weight). If the diagnosis is confirmed, the child should be put on a lactose-free milk substitute for at least six weeks and then the challenge repeated. This approach is quite different from the all-too-common practice of simply putting the child on a soya milk for an indefinite period without a proper diagnosis being made.

Which lactose-free milk substitute should be used? In straightforward lactose deficiency, the relatively inexpensive soya milk substitutes (for example Wysoy) are all that is needed. Some authorities would advocate using a much more expensive semi-synthetic milk, such as Pregestimil, the argument being that, if cow's milk protein allergy is present, the child is quite likely also to develop an allergy to soya protein. However, we have already said that cow's milk protein allergy is extremely rare and, in the authors' experience, this is not a problem. If, at the end of six weeks, when milk products are reintroduced, the child is still symptomatic, or if symptoms persist on a soya preparation, the child should be referred to a paediatrician.

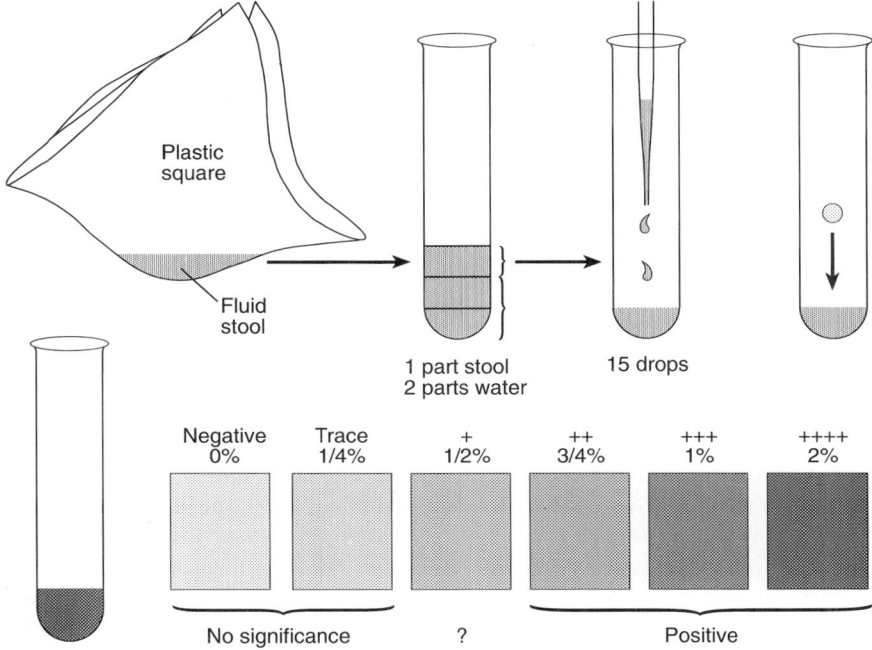

Figure 4.2 Test for lactose (reducing substances) in stool using Ames Clinitest tablet.

OTHER CAUSES OF PERSISTENT DIARRHOEA IN CHILDREN

We have just discussed children with persistent diarrhoea following acute gastroenteritis. Other children of all ages are brought to the general practitioner with a complaint that they have persistent or chronic diarrhoea. Make sure you clarify exactly what is meant. The term 'chronic' to some people indicates severity rather than duration and many people do not understand that there is a wide range of normal bowel habit. For example, a healthy breast-fed baby may produce several small loose stools each day or may not have his or her bowels open at all for several days. An older child may have three soft bowel movements a day, which can be as normal as having bowel movements every second day. Parents may worry about the colour of the child's stool—green being particularly alarming, although in an otherwise well child, it has no significance. The word 'diarrhoea' refers to the abnormal consistency of a stool rather than its frequency, though usually, but not invariably, stool frequency is increased.

For practical purposes, we can consider diarrhoea as originating either from the small bowel or the large bowel. Most diarrhoeas presenting in general practice originate in the large bowel. They result from rapid transit of the stool through the colon so that less water is reabsorbed and the stool is watery, although otherwise normal. Diarrhoea arising from the small bowel however has implications of malabsorption. If the small bowel is malfunctioning, substances which would have normally been absorbed, such as fats, pass on into the colon where they may ferment and putrify and the resulting diarrhoea is offensive, bulky, fatty, and may be accompanied by excessive flatus. Because of the loss of essential nutrients, chronic small bowel diarrhoea is associated with failure to thrive and deficiency states.

The most common chronic diarrhoea of childhood which presents to a general practitioner is the so-called 'toddler diarrhoea' or 'peas and carrots syndrome'. This is a large bowel diarrhoea. As the name suggests, a young child passes frequent stools in which food particles are easily identified. Fluid ileocaecal contents are virtually emptied out of the rectum and down the legs at inconvenient times. The mother is worried because she cannot potty train the child and the playgroup will not take him or her. The stool pattern is variable, the child is thriving and his or her appetite is good. The identifiable food particles do not represent malabsorption. Cellulose-containing foods, such as peas or sweetcorn, may be present in all stools but, usually, the firm consistency of a stool masks them. Toddler diarrhoea may represent one end of a spectrum of colonic sensitivity. It may be helpful when explaining the condition to the parents to describe the child as having a very sensitive colon which responds over-vigorously to such stimuli as infection, stress, excitement, and natural laxatives occurring in the diet. Given time, these childrens' colons seem to settle down and there is no evidence that they will have irritable bowel syndrome as adults. In practice, the symptoms usually resolve by school entry age.

Presented with an obviously well child giving a history suggestive of toddler diarrhoea and having established on the child's growth chart that there is no evidence of failure to thrive, one can explain the situation to the mother, point out that the child is well, discuss the likely cause, and suggest that she returns in a few weeks, having kept a diary showing diet and occurrence of diarrhoea. The diary may show that the child's diet contains many natural laxatives. Blackcurrant juice, other fruit juices, raisins, and other dried fruit are often implicated. The authors have seen children whose problem resolved when their intake of blackcurrant juice was reduced from several bottlefuls a day. The diary may also show clear emotional triggers for the diarrhoea, which can be discussed with the mother. Dietary modification may be indicated, but the general practitioner should avoid the trap of discussing food allergies which may take the situation into a completely different realm and medicalize it unnecessarily. There is absolutely no place for symptomatic treatment. Remember that the problem is largely a social one of embarassment for the parents, rather than a symptomatic one for the child. As such, it deserves to be followed up by the general practitioner or health visitor, and if at any time there is evidence that the child is failing to thrive he or she should be referred.

Coeliac disease and cystic fibrosis

Coeliac disease and cystic fibrosis are very uncommon causes of persisent diarrhoea in children, but they will be discussed here briefly because they illustrate several important points. Children with these conditions have characteristic small bowel diarrhoea. In cystic fibrosis, this results from maldigestion because of pancreatic insufficiency but the absorption process is normal. In coeliac disease, the digestive process is normal but there is malabsorption. These children are not thriving and an important diagnostic tool for the general practitioner is the weight chart (see Fig. 4.3). The child with coeliac disease is miserable, anorexic, and has a bloated stomach and flat buttocks. He or she is anaemic and occasionally, paradoxically, constipated. The cystic child is quite lively. He or she also may have a bloated stomach and there will usually be other clues to the diagnosis, such as chest infections. The clinical pictures are usually clear-cut but, occasionally, it might be possible to confuse the two conditions. The fundamental point to make in a general practice context is that any child with a chronic small bowel diarrhoea who is not thriving, should be referred immediately for investigation. There is absolutely no place, either in general practice or in hospital practice, for the trial of a gluten-free diet

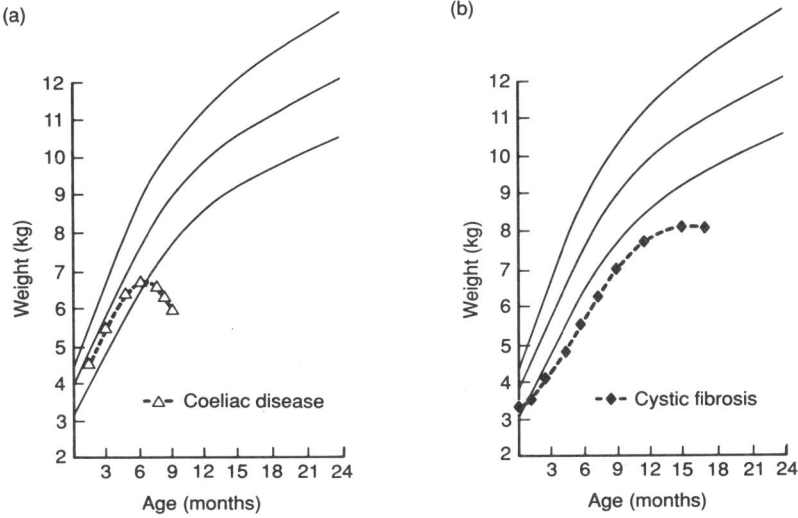

Fig. 4.3 Classical growth charts (weight) in (a) coeliac disease and (b) cystic fibrosis.

in the absence of a proper diagnosis, although unfortunately, this still occurs.

THE CHILD WHO IS CONSTIPATED

Constipation can be regarded as delayed or incomplete passage of stool sufficient to cause a child or his or her parents distressing symptoms. As stated previously, bowel habit has a wide range of normality. We must make sure that a complaint of constipation in a child is not the parents' abnormal perception of what bowel habit 'ought to be'. Normality is not determined by frequency of defecation, but by the complete emptying of the rectum on a regular basis. For some people this happens normally every three or four days, for others it happens two or three times a day. Most constipation in children is short-term and acute and is dealt with by their parents. However, if stool is chronically retained a chain of events is set in motion. The colon and rectum lose their tone. The gastrocolic reflex causes discomfort, resulting in complaints of vague abdominal pain after food and the child unconsciously begins to select a low-residue diet and becomes anorexic. As the stool becomes harder, the child is more and more reluctant to defecate. Liquid stool is still entering the colon through the ileocaecal valve and, in advanced cases, will percolate around the large mass of stool in the colon and rectum and present as liquid faecal soiling. Parents bringing their children to the doctor with this 'spurious diarrhoea' may be angry with the child for loss of control and incredulous when the doctor suggests that this is due to constipation. The distended colon may press on the bladder, causing enuresis or even urinary retention with infection.

The history can be difficult because most parents stop being interested in their child's bowel habit once he or she can go to the lavatory alone. However, time spent on a history is important because, not infrequently, emotional factors are found to underlie the condition or to have developed subsequently. Sometimes the problem seems to have started from a specific incident, such as a hospital admission for minor surgery or a single episode of painful defecation, perhaps with a small fissure. It may have started in a child who has unpleasant associations with defecation, such as too rigorous or too early potty training. In an older child, unpleasant school lavatories may be the cause. Sometimes children consciously or unconsciously use their bowel actions to manipulate their families, for example, when they feel displaced and wish to emphasize their existence, perhaps because there is a new sibling in the family or their parents are fighting each other.

We have described a developing picture and children may present to the general practitioner at any point with any of the symptoms described, not only with infrequent passage of stools but with abdominal pain, especially after meals, enuresis, urinary tract infection, faecal soiling, or screaming when taken near the toilet or potty. If this condition is recognized early a lot of misery can be avoided.

If constipation is suspected, try to examine the child lying down. Sometimes the abdomen is obviously distended and hard masses, like potatoes, are felt in the transverse and descending colon. Sometimes a mass, like a pregnant uterus, is felt coming out of the pelvis. Should these children have a rectal examination? This is very debatable and we must all make up our own minds. Certainly, the anus should be gently inspected to look for a fissure, remembering that a child with chronic constipation may have reflex anal dilatation. If the child is going to be referred on, it is probably not justified to submit him or her to a rectal examination, which will almost certainly be repeated by the paediatrician. However, if the doctor feels confident in him or herself and in the situation, a gentle rectal examination can be very helpful. An abdominal mass may not have been felt, so a rectum full of craggy stool helps to confirm the diagnosis. In the presence of a distended abdomen, rectal examination, which reveals a tight anal canal and an empty rectum, could point to the extrememly rare condition of Hirschsprung's disease, and the child should be referred immediately.

Management aims to empty the rectum and then to help the family establish a regular pattern of emptying. How the initial emptying is carried out will depend on the stage of the constipation, the doctor's experience, and the availability of suitably trained nursing help. In early or moderate cases, stimulant laxatives, such as senna, may be all that is needed. Bulking laxatives, such as lactulose or Fybogel, should not be given until the retained faeces have been cleared. The senna is started in small doses and titrated according to the child's individual needs. For example, a moderately constipated 3-year-old can be given 5 ml of senna syrup nightly, increasing every second night by 5 ml until diarrhoea is produced, at which stage faecal 'rocks' are also passed. The required dose of senna is very individual and may be as much as 25 or 30 ml per day. The main risk of overdose is severe colic and this can be avoided if the dose is given incrementally.

Once diarrhoea is produced the senna is reduced and adjusted to produce a formed or semi-formed stool each day. In more advanced cases it may be necessary to empty the rectum with an enema on two consecutive days and then to institute senna. Repeated enemas and suppositories must be avoided and, if the doctor is not confident that he or she is coping with the initial emptying quickly, the child should be referred.

If the child establishes a regular emptying pattern, regular senna should be maintained and the diet modified to contain sufficient bulk. Some children cannot be persuaded to eat vegetables, fruit, and bran, so it may be necessary to use lactulose in addition to senna. The senna is given nightly and very regularly; the lactulose is given twice daily. As the child's bowel tone returns, the reduced need for laxatives will become self-evident, but it may be necessary to keep up the laxatives for many months. There is absolutely no place for the use of other laxatives, such as liquid paraffin, phenolphthalein, or osmotic salts in children.

We have described an approach to the physical problems of constipation, but we have also pointed out that there are frequently associated emotional problems and these should be looked for by the doctor or health visitor. Most of these problems will respond to a common sense approach by an outsider who has not become embroiled in the family disturbance. Referral to a child guidance clinic is hardly ever necessary.

Very small unweaned infants are quite often brought to the doctor with a complaint that their stools are extremely hard and that they pass them with great difficulty. The mother is distressed and may have had to help the stools out. Most of these babies are well and thriving. Physical examination is quite normal and it is important to make sure that there really is a problem for the baby and that it is not just the mother's perception which needs reassurance. At this age, the problem is usually not long-lasting. It might be regarded, like colic, as an immaturity of gut motility. Make sure that the baby is having sufficient fluid. Do not suggest diluting milk feeds but advise additional clear fluids between bottles or breast-feeds. It may be worth trying the old-fashioned remedy of brown sugar, which acts rather like lactulose. If all else fails, a small dose of lactulose will help or, if the baby is already weaned, small amounts of puréed fruit may be given. Paediatric glycerine suppositories may very occasionally be required. Congenital abnormalities, such as Hirschsprung's disease, causing constipation, are very rare. Babies with Hirschsprung's disease present with abdominal distention, constipation, and are not thriving. They should be referred immediately.

THE CHILD WITH RECURRENT ABDOMINAL PAIN

Colic

A thriving baby is often brought to the doctor or health visitor by the mother with the complaint that he or she screams, pulls up his or her knees, and passes large amounts of wind, often in the evenings. A diagnosis of colic can confidently be made. No one knows what causes colic, though there are many theories, such as poorly developed peristalsis, food allergy, lactose intolerance, and poor feeding technique. It is allegedly almost unknown in France and the observation that it is less common in large families and more common in first babies, lends support to the theory that there is a strong parental perceptual element. Colic is self-limiting and has no known sequelae, providing the baby avoids being battered by his or her distraught parents, because we should not underestimate the disruption this condition can cause. It is therefore important to spend time listening to the parents and to examine the child carefully. No treatment is known to cure colic, but traditional therapies seem to help a little. Many parents have often tried medication before they finally come to the doctor and some proprietary remedies may help because of their alcohol content. Given the benign course of colic, it is important that, whatever else the doctor does, he or she should do no harm. Changing milk brands or instituting soya milk is not justified. Some infants, who may be air swallowers, may be helped by advice on feeding position, changing teat design and flow rate, and altering feeding frequency. Infant Gaviscon may occasionally be helpful. The support of a good health visitor and other mothers who have been through the same situation is probably more helpful than anything else. Be aware that repeated consultations may be a cry for help from a mother who is not coping and who is depressed.

The older child with recurrent abdominal pain

Recurrent abdominal pain is a very common reason for children to present to their general practitioner. It is very difficult to assess because it is such a subjective complaint and, frequently, there is no objective way of knowing its true severity or cause. Organic causes are very rare. Constipation can present as recurrent abdominal pain, as we have already discussed, and urinary tract pathology must always be considered. Peptic ulceration, either in the stomach, duodenum or Meckel's diverticulum, cholelithiasis, lead poisoning, Henoch–Schönlein purpura, and liver disease are all very rare causes of recurrent abdominal pain in children and there will usually be some additional features which make the general practitioner realize that something more serious is going on and that the child needs referral. A particularly interested general practitioner might like to investigate for these conditions; full blood count, erythrocyte sedimentation rate, liver function tests, and abdominal ultrasound may be helpful.

Emotional factors are often unearthed in these children and their families. Whether or not these emotional factors are cause or effect is debatable, and there is a vast literature on the subject. It is true to say that recurrent abdominal pain may be more frequent in more intelligent 'sensitive' children, and parents are often very reassured by this observation. A group of these children will go on to develop adult-type migraine and these often show the classical personality characteristics of perfectionism, rigidity, and the setting of high personal goals. Recurrent abdominal pain may be the presenting symptom of more serious psychosocial pathology, such as sexual abuse. A rare, but interesting, condition is the syndrome of Munchausen by proxy. In this situation, the child's symptoms are trivial but there is some gain for the parents in having a child with symptoms and there may be great pressure to have the child investigated and to have a variety of invasive tests and complex treatments.

Management will start with a good history and examination including measurement of height and weight. Constipation will be excluded. It may help parents if you explain that diagnoses, such as 'little bellyachers', 'billiousness', 'abdominal migraine', and 'recurrent abdominal migraine of childhood' reflect the long historical pedigree of these symptoms and that they have a lack of precise explanation or guaranteed cure. An allegedly high frequency of symptoms is often put into a much more modest perspective if the parents are asked to keep a diary of the pain over a period of several weeks. The diary should include severity of pain, duration, time of occurrence, and associated events. The exclusion of sinister pathology, along with the sympathetic approach to the child and parents, will almost certainly produce an improvement that will be apparent in the diary. Identification of obvious stress factors from the diary, for example that the pain is worse before certain school events, or before visits to an estranged parent, may point to opportunities for social manipulation. In the absence of identifiable pathology there is absolutely no place for drug treatment, and management should be directed towards changing the perceptions of the family and behaviour modification in the child. Continuing review, using the diary, showing obvious pleasure and praise for increasing 'good patches' will allow the child to feel that he or she has some control over his or her symptoms and this usually helps. If after trying this management, symptoms do not abate or are sufficient to disrupt normal functioning in a school or home setting, then referral should be considered.

THE CHILD WITH BLOOD IN THE STOOLS

A parent finding blood in a child's stools is understandably frightened. In practice there is seldom a sinister pathology, particularly if the bleeding only occurs once or several times over a few days. In most cases no cause is found and the bleeding is probably coming from a small fissure or internal tear. An obvious anal fissure may be seen and constipation should be looked for. In a breast-fed child the blood may be coming from the mother. Sometimes a mother may be found to have a cracked nipple with blood in her expressed milk.

Recurrent or continuous rectal bleeding may have a serious cause. Colonic polyps or inflammatory bowel disease may first present with rectal bleeding. Cow's milk protein allergy, intussusception due to Henoch–

Schölein purpura and sexual abuse may all produce blood in the stools but other symptoms will usually predominate. Any child in whom rectal bleeding persists with no good explanation should be referred.

INFLAMMATORY BOWEL DISEASE

Inflammatory bowel disease is very rare in childhood and the pattern is quite different from that seen in adults, although in the early teens the distinctive adult patterns of ulcerative colitis and Crohn's disease begin to emerge. Children may present with chronic diarrhoea with blood and mucus, recurrent abdominal pain, and be found to have a raised erythrocyte sedimentation rate. Clinically and histologically there may not be a distinction between Crohn's disease and ulcerative colitis in the younger child and the likelihood of recovery is much greater than in adults. This is a condition which requires shared care with the specialist.

THE JAUNDICED BABY

Physiological jaundice is universal and may produce anything between an imperceptible rise in bilirubin and an obviously jaundiced baby who may require phototherapy or even, very occasionally, exchange transfusion. Diagnostic problems arise when the apparently physiological jaundice persists beyond the first week of life, or where jaundice appears for the first time after the first week. The general practitioner has to ask him or herself whether this is due to a prolongation of physiological jaundice due to relative underfeeding, whether the child has breast milk jaundice, whether the child has an infection, or whether the child could possibly have one of any number of very rare congenital conditions (see Fig. 4.1) which could be disastrous if missed. In this context the most important of these conditions for the general practitioner to consider are probably biliary atresia and neonatal hepatitis.

Breast milk jaundice is non-progressive. The child is well, feeding and functioning normally. The bilirubin remains stable and is predominantly conjugated. The diagnosis can be confirmed by stopping breast-feeding for a couple of days and the bilirubin will invariably fall. Unfortunately, the use of formula milk in this situation negates one of the arguments for breast-feeding, i.e. the avoidance of foreign protein. Breast milk jaundice may continue for months and has no sequelae. Intrauterine infections, such as toxoplasmosis, herpes, cytomegalovirus, and rubella can also present with neonatal jaundice, but there are usually other indicators such as hepatomegaly. Acute infections acquired postnatally, commonly urinary tract infections, can also present with jaundice and urinalysis must be part of first-line investigations of a jaundiced baby. Two of the most sinister causes of jaundice in the neonate, biliary atresia and neonatal hepatitis, may present with jaundice in a child who appears to be otherwise quite well, and the danger is that these children will not be referred early enough for effective treatment. If surgery for biliary atresia is delayed beyond six weeks the prognosis is very poor. This emphasizes the fundamental importance of making a clear diagnosis of neonatal jaundice well before the sixth week of life. If there are any doubts, or if the baby presents late, the general practitioner should refer immediately.

FURTHER READING

General paediatric and paediatric gastroenterology textbooks

All the current textbooks cover these subjects well. They are all being upgraded and there is no particular reason to recommend one more than any of the others for general reading.

Insley, J. (ed.) (1990). *A paediatric vade-mecum*, (13th ed). Lloyd-Luke (Medical Books), London.

This is a gold-mine of factual information, which includes growth chart, blood values, dosages, and recommended emergency management of the whole range of paediatric conditions, including gastroenterological ones.

Selected monographs

Apley, J. (1959). *The child with abdominal pains*. Blackwell Scientific Publications, Oxford.
Clayden, G. S. (1991). Constipation. In *Recent advances in paediatrics*, **9**, pp. 41–59. Churchill Livingstone, London.
Costello, A. and Bhutta, T. (1992). Antidiarrhoeal drugs for acute diarrhoea in children. *British Medical Journal*, **304**, 1–2.
Michener, W. M. and Wyllie, R. (1990). Management of children and adolescents with inflammatory bowel disease. *Medical Clinics of North America*, **74**.

5 Gastrointestinal disorders in the elderly

Sanjeebit Jachuck and Oliver James

Gastroenterology in the elderly is an important subject; the gastrointestinal organs undergo morphological, histological, and functional changes with advancing age and some of these changes underlie characteristic clinical presentations that signify the aging gut. The natural history of a number of common conditions seen in younger individuals may be quite different in old age. Advancing age is also associated with an increase in morbidity and increased use of medication, both of which can affect the gut.

Gastrointestinal diseases are commonly encountered in older patients and make a heavy demand on primary care and hospital services. In a study undertaken in North America, gastrointestinal problems accounted for 18 per cent of all patients attending a geriatric clinic, 27 per cent of all hospital admissions, and 20 per cent of geriatric deaths. In the UK 50 per cent of acute medical and surgical beds are occupied by older patients. Not surprisingly the subject is attracting growing interest, although at the same time there is a demand to rationalize our use of hospital resources.

The size of the ageing community in the UK is progressively increasing. At present, approximately 17 per cent of the population are above 65 years of age. It is predicted that over the next two decades the number of people over the age of 75 years will increase by 23 per cent and the number over the age of 85 years will increase by 42 per cent. Most elderly people live at home, and the effort to keep them there will fall largely on family doctors.

THE SPECTRUM OF GASTROINTESTINAL PROBLEMS IN THE ELDERLY

In a recent questionnaire survey of 2066 individuals in Southampton, dyspepsia was reported in 37 per cent of women and 31 per cent of men aged between 70 and 79 years. In patients aged over 80 years dyspepsia was reported by 24 per cent of women and 4 per cent of men. A study of 594 consecutive people aged over 70 years, registered with a group practice in Newcastle upon Tyne, revealed the range of gastrointestinal diagnoses made in the elderly in general practice (Table 5.1). About 20 per cent had significant conditions related to the upper gastrointestinal tract, and 75 per cent of older individuals with symptoms were found, on investigation, to have positive pathology, with over 80 per cent of these conditions related

Table 5.1 *Gastrointestinal problems in the elderly (n = 594)*

	Men		Women		
	70–74 years	> 75 years	70–74 years	> 75 years	
Gastrointestinal problem	(n = 122)	(n = 75)	(n = 162)	(n = 235)	Total
Dyspepsia	2	2	4	9	17
Hiatus hernia	6	2	12	6	26
Gastritis	—	—	1	3	4
Gastric ulcer	2	2	7	6	17
Duodenal ulcer	8	1	4	5	18
Gastrointestinal surgery	3	2	6	9	20
Diverticular disease	4	1	5	8	18
Carcinoma of the rectum	—	1	1	—	2
Rectal surgery	—	1	1	—	2
Total	25	12	41	46	124

(Adapted from Jachuck, S. (1988). *Evaluation of the need in care of the elderly in a general practice*. Medical Research Centre, Newcastle upon Tyne.)

to the upper gastrointestinal tract. This morbidity pattern is similar to that seen in younger people, but the clinical manifestations of these conditions and their management are often different in old age. For example, elderly patients with peptic ulcer disease do not always complain of pain and, conversely, those over 70 years of age frequently report a variety of abdominal symptoms suggestive of colorectal cancer, but these may merely be manifestations of the ageing and failing gut. (Table 5.2).

The incidence of most diseases increases with age, and many conditions

Table 5.2 *Bowel symptoms observed in a sample of the community in Newcastle Upon Tyne*

	Age		
Symptoms	< 70 years	> 70 years	p value
Abdominal pain	4	11	< 0.05
Mucus per rectum	2	10	< 0.01
Faecal incontinence	0	6	< 0.05
Change in flatus	8	17	< 0.05
Malaise	17	32	< 0.05
Anorexia	3	11	< 0.05
Bloating	11	22	< 0.05

(Adapted from Curless, R., French, J. M., Williams, G., and James, O. F. W. (1991). A comparison of the frequency of bowel symptoms in young and old community controls versus colorectal carcinoma patients. Presented at the British Geriatric Society Scientific Meeting, London, October 1991.)

such as rheumatoid arthritis, vascular disease, and diabetes mellitus, directly or indirectly affect the gastrointestinal tract. These conditions may affect the mucosa or influence gut motility and may cause bleeding or gastroparesis. In certain neuromuscular disorders, such as cerebrovascular diseases, Parkinsonism, multiple sclerosis, polymyositis, systemic sclerosis, and motor neurone disease, gastrointestinal disorders such as dysphagia are not uncommon.

A large proportion of elderly people receive medication which may contribute to disorders of the gut. Mechanisms include a direct mucosal effect, producing inflammatory changes or impaired permeability, impaired motility leading to altered transit time, lack of protective prostaglandins, and altered bowel flora. Therapeutic effects may be amplified because of impaired renal clearance, hepatic dysfunction, and through drug interaction. Many old people self-medicate with drugs, such as aspirin, laxatives and other over-the-counter medication, which also affect the gut. Some of the commonly prescribed medications and their effects are listed in Table 5.3.

Table 5.3 *Drugs affecting the gastrointestinal tract*

Manifestations	Pathology	Drugs attributed
Oral lesions	Gingivitis, ulceration, Lichen planus, candidiasis	Phenytoin, nifedipine, non-steroidal anti-inflammatory drugs, beta-blocking drugs, inhaled steroids, cytotoxic drugs
Dyspepsia	Inflammation, ulceration	Non-steroidal anti-inflammatory drugs, digoxin, potassium Chloride, ferrous sulphate, antibiotics, oestrogen, opioid drugs
Bleeding and pain	Ulceration and bleeding	Non-steroidal anti-inflammatory drugs, slow-release potassium chloride, corticosteroids, tetracycline, phenolphthalein
Malabsorption	Alteration of intestinal flora, mucosal injury, cellular changes	Tetracycline, phenytoin, phenobarbitone, Biguanides, metformin, mefenamic acid, cytotoxic drugs, cholestyramine, *P*-aminosalicylic acid
Constipation	Ileus	Tricyclic antidepressants, anti-Parkinsonian drugs, chlorpromazine, anticholinergic drugs, morphine, ferrous sulphate, certain antacids
Diarrhoea	Motility disorder	Digoxin, thyroxine, laxatives, magnesium-containing antacids, antibiotics

It is important to make a special mention of non-steroidal anti-inflammatory drugs (NSAIDs). Haematemesis, melaena or ulcer perforation occur 3–4 times more commonly in patients taking these drugs compared with controls. More than 24 million prescriptions for NSAIDs are dispensed every year in the UK, and most are for the elderly. Patients over 60 years of age are at increased risk of complications and mortality rises considerably with increasing age. The drugs affect the mucosal defence mechanisms by interfering with the integrity and synthesis of mucus, bicarbonate secretion, synthesis of cytoprotective prostaglandins, pepsinogen activation, and pepsin release. They also affect stomach blood flow, intestinal permeability, and cause small bowel blood loss, ulceration, and stricture formation.

Levels of alcohol consumption are also increasing in this age group. A random sample study of 241 elderly people in London revealed that 51 per cent of men and 22 per cent of women reported drinking alcohol in the previous three months, and 35 per cent of all drinkers reported drinking alcohol each day. Although the majority of the individuals studied remained within the 'safe' limit, the possible contribution of alcohol to gastrointestinal problems should be borne in mind.

PATHOPHYSIOLOGICAL CHANGES IN THE GASTROINTESTINAL TRACT

Four main types of pathophysiological changes are associated with old age:

(1) cellular changes;
(2) functional changes for example motility, secretory, metabolism;
(3) vascular changes;
(4) neoplasia.

Cellular changes

Progressive loss of teeth is a common feature of old age. Irregular teeth cause damage to gums and oral mucosa. Infection of gums and teeth also affects mastication. Progressive loss of acinar cells and fibrosis of the salivary glands reduces secretion. Certain disease conditions, such as sicca syndrome, also affect secretory activities. Trauma and decreased salivary secretion lead to oral ulceration, inflammation, and infection of buccal mucosa, as well as affecting digestion and absorption of food. Some systemic diseases and drugs are associated with mucosal lesions, such as lichen planus, gingivitis, and oral candidiasis.

Cellular changes in the oesophagus seen in older individuals are usually due to long-standing inflammatory conditions which result in fibrosis, shortening of the gullet, and stricture formation. Anoxic changes affecting flexibility and tensile strength of collagen may result in Zenker's diverticulum. Columnar epithelium in the distal oesophagus is reported in up to 20 per cent of individuals with endoscopic evidence of oesophagitis. This is called Barrett's oesophagus and is a pre-malignant condition associated with the development of adenocarcinoma.

Chronic gastritis and gastric atrophy are common with increasing age; these are thought by some to be disease processes and not simply consequences of ageing. Autoimmune, hypersecretory, and environmental factors have been suggested as contributing causes. In a study of gastric biopsies from 201 elderly subjects, gastric atrophy was observed in most specimens. In later life, large gastric folds are often found in the stomach. They usually remain unchanged, but in some individuals they increase in size.

Helicobacter pylori is a common pathogen considered to contribute to chronic gastritis and relapse of peptic ulcer. The organism is found in more than 50 per cent of healthy, asymptomatic individuals and the prevalence of the infection increases by 10 per cent per decade in the community. It is twice as common in Black people. The presence of *Helicobacter pylori* in the elderly was found to have a close association with the presence of duodenal ulcer. The infection was not associated with use of NSAIDs, H_2 inhibitors, alcohol or tobacco. It has been suggested that in all elderly patients with duodenal ulcer and *Helicobacter pylori*, attempts should be made to treat the infection.

Characteristic histological changes in the small intestine are seen with advancing age. The changes affect villi and surface area. There is an increase in leaf-shaped, broad villi, and parallel ridges. There is a concurrent reduction in villous height and significant reduction in surface area. Such changes are thought to be due to reduced cell production in the mucosa and may be linked to impaired absorption. Similar but reversible histological changes have been reported following bacterial overgrowth. In duodenal biopsy specimens from elderly patients with bacterial overgrowth there is significant loss of villi and crypt depth. There are greater numbers of leaf-shaped villi and convolutions. These changes are likely to be due to increased shedding of surface epithelium through bacterial action. Details of degenerative changes detected by electron microscopy include changes in the microvilli, disruption of terminal webs, and swelling of mitochondria and endoplasmic reticulum. Such histological changes revert when bacteria are eliminated or reduced in number in response to therapy. It is likely that these histological changes in the small bowel associated with bacterial overgrowth are a significant cause of malabsorption in older people.

Increased gastrointestinal infection in older people may be due to a decline in secretory mucosal immune function in the gut's lymphoid system associated with advancing age. However, when production of immuno-globulins by the duodenal mucosa in patients aged 70 years or older is compared with that of patients aged 50 years or younger, only marginal differences have been found between the two groups, suggesting that ageing may not have a major effect of duodenal mucosal immune mechanisms.

DIVERTICULOSIS: IS IT A DISEASE?

Diverticulosis is uncommon in individuals under the age of 40 years. It is a condition of ageing and may affect 30 per cent of the population over the age of 60 years and 66 per cent of the population over the age of 80 years. It is usually confined to the sigmoid colon and occurs more commonly in white people. It is claimed to be less common in vegetarians. The changes seen in the bowel are muscle thickening, cell hypertrophy, and shortening of the colon. Episodic inflammation may be seen in these diverticula. Recurrent episodes may lead to fibrosis, stricture, adhesion, and fistula formation. Bleeding due to erosion of vessels occurs in about 15 per cent of patients with the condition. Anaemia in patients with duodenal diverticular disease has also been reported. There is no causal relationship between diverticular disease and cancer of the colon, but the condition is undoubtedly a cause of substantial morbidity in older people.

FUNCTIONAL CHANGES

Increasing age is associated with some alteration of gastric emptying, although this is of doubtful clinical significance. Acid and pepsin secretion decrease with advancing age and the incidence of achlorhydria increases. Pathological gastro-oesophageal reflux is common in old people and is due to impaired lower oesophageal sphincter function. Hiatus hernia, both sliding and para-oesophageal, increases in incidence with age, although it is not a major factor predisposing to reflux.

Pathophysiological changes in the gut may cause malabsorption in up to 13 per cent of old people. Poor carbohydrate, fat, and protein absorption may also be due to inadequate diet in these patients. However, malabsorption of iron, folate, vitamin B12, and calcium are common in this age group. Certain drugs, such as antibiotics, anticonvulsants, and laxatives, if used in excess, can also contribute to malabsorption. It is not easy to diagnose the condition as these patients are often without symptoms. The most common manifestations are malaise, weight loss or anaemia, and the laboratory investigations used to establish the diagnosis are similar to those used in younger adults.

Constipation is the most common gastrointestinal disorder in the UK. People suffer from constipation more frequently as they get older. Normal colonic activity is responsible for mixing the contents of the stool and co-ordinating peristalsis which propels the stools distally. Dietary components, such as carbohydrate, protein, and fibre, are the most important local factors regulating colonic function. Impaired mobility, difficulty in assuming an upright posture or undertaking exercise also contribute to the condition. Poor dentition with decreased production of saliva, inadequate intake of fibre, lack of variety of food, and lack of urge to defecate are other contributory factors. Balance between sympathetic and para-sympathetic activity is an important factor. Certain metabolic disorders (for example hypercalcaemia), endocrine disorders (for example hypo-thyroidism and diabetes mellitus), chronic renal failure, neurological conditions, depression, and adenocarcinoma of the colon are often associated with constipation. Certain drugs (listed in Table 5.3) are known to cause constiptation and faecal impaction. This problem accounted for 42 per cent of admissions to the geriatric wards of a district hospital during one year.

Diarrhoea is almost as common as constipation and can paradoxically be due to constipation with overflow. It is usually due to infection, intolerance to certain fatty foods, overindulgence in laxatives, and following antibiotic therapy. Spurious diarrhoea or retention with overflow is seen in constipated patients with faecal impaction. Organic causes of diarrhoea include diverticular disease, inflammatory bowel disease, malabsorption, malignancy, post-gastrectomy syndrome, and other conditions affecting motility. Bacterial contamination of the bowel is the most common cause of diarrhoea in this age group.

Faecal incontinence is a major problem in the care of older patients. In long-stay geriatric wards, faecal incontinence was found in 45 per cent of patients. In residential homes, it occurs in approximately 10 per cent of residents. These patients were also found to have bacteruria. This may be due to a weakness of the urethral sphincter seen in pudendal neuropathy.

VASCULAR CHANGES

Progressive atheromatous changes are commonly associated with advancing age. Such changes interfere with the normal vascular response to bleeding and may account for difficulty in controlling bleeding from gastrointestinal lesions in the elderly. Inflammatory diseases, occlusive and non-occlusive infarction, and venous disorders all contribute to the pathogenesis of ischaemic bowel disease. Any decompensation in cardiac output also adversely affects the gastrointestinal mucosa and organs as the splanchinic circulation normally receives the largest fraction of the cardiac output. Ischaemic bowel disorder should be considered in elderly individuals with unexplained abdominal pain, blood-stained diarrhoea, and pseudo-obstruction, particularly if they have clinical evidence of arteriopathy, cardiac dysrhythmia, and/or decompensation.

NEOPLASIA

Primary neoplasm and metastatic involvement of the gastrointestinal tract is very common and it is also a common cause of death in the elderly. Malignant changes are also seen in association with certain pre-existing diseases of the gastrointestinal tract. Malignant transformation of gastric ulcer is probably very common; patients with extensive ulcerative colitis and Crohn's disease are also at risk of developing malignancy. Lymphomas can occur in association with coeliac disease. Risk of developing cancer is high in metaplastic polyps of colon, particularly those more than 20 mm in diameter. By the time patients present to their general practitioner with clinical manifestation of these diseases, the pathology is often advanced and although diagnostic delay may influence prognosis, progression of neoplasms in very old people is often remarkably slow. The most common benign neoplasms of the small intestine and colon are polyps, adenomas, lipomas, and haemangioma. They also can present with obstruction and haemorrhage.

COMMON DISEASES

Peptic ulcer

Peptic ulcer disease affects 10 per cent of the male population in Western society at some stage of life. A general practitioner with a list size of 2500 patients will have approximately 12 new patients with peptic ulcer disease per year and 125 patients who have had the disease. Although the exact incidence of the disease in the elderly community is not well documented, it is reported that the age-specific incidence of the disease progressively increases with age up to the age of 80 years. There has been a steady decline in the male to female ratio in peptic ulcer disease and although gastric ulcer remains twice as common in men as women, the sex ratio for duodenal ulcer disease is approaching unity. Presenting symptoms are often atypical. Pain is less freqently the initial complaint in this age group. Pain, when present, may be uncharacteristic and its relation to food can be vague and inconsistent. Melaena can be a common presentation of the disease. Patients may even present with anorexia, weight loss, malaise, or angina secondary to anaemia. Ulcer complications, such as haemorrhage and perforation, can be the presenting symptoms. There may be little in the way of objective clinical findings except in cases of haemorrhage and perforation.

The disease is a chronic condition and relapses periodically. Smoking, stress, drugs, infection, and pathophysiological changes associated with the ageing process may contribute to the aetiology, relapse, and complications. A high degree of suspicion and an effective surveillance plan is important to detect the disease early, control the condition, and contain the complications to modify morbidity and mortality.

In a study of the outcome of peptic ulcer in the elderly, the overall cumulative rate of ulcer haemorrhage, perforation or related death was found to be 19 per cent. Women had a greater rate than the men (women 21 per cent, men 14 per cent). A retrospective hospital study of duodenal ulcer disease in the elderly revealed that 80 per cent of the patients were admitted with acute complications, 50 per cent with haemorrhage, and 30 per cent with perforation. It is reported that 80 per cent of all ulcer deaths occur in those aged 65 years or over and 85 per cent of all ulcers needing surgical attention are in patients over 75 years of age.

Early diagnosis and prompt intervention is essential in the management of peptic ulcer disease in the elderly. Endoscopy is the investigation preferred by most clinicians in the elderly. It is safe and frequently produces useful information. It enables the clinician to detect ulcers, record any suspicious morphological appearances, and obtain biopsies for histological evaluation. It is also capable of distinguishing duodenal scarring from active ulceration. In one report endoscopic examination undertaken in patients over 70 years of age revealed significant abnormalities in two-thirds of the patients and influenced future management in the remaining one-third. Radiology is useful in defining anatomical structure beyond a stenotic lesion and it is suggested that a barium swallow should be mandatory in patients with dysphagia before undertaking endoscopic examination to exclude high oesophageal pathology.

Management is no different from that in the younger patients. Histamine-2 receptor antagonists remain the drugs of choice. There is little to choose between cimetidine and ranitidine. Permanent maintenance therapy is considered to be a safer option in elderly patients. A confusional state occasionally develops in the older patients receiving cimetidine, related to impaired renal function. Those with larger ulcers may require more aggresive therapy and for a longer period. Misoprostol, a prostaglandin E1 analogue, is claimed to prevent and heal NSAID-induced ulceration while the patient continues to take the NSAID. Side-effects can be a problem and co-prescription of an H_2-receptor antagonist with an NSAID may be equally effective. A prospective study of duodenal ulcer admissions suggested early endoscopic diagnosis, adequate resuscitation, and early elective surgery are necessary to reduce mortality following complications. An American study of emergency management of perforated peptic ulcer in patients of 60 years of age or older recommend gastrectomy for perforated gastric ulcer, and truncal vagotomy and hemigastrectomy for perforated duodenal ulcer as the operative procedures with best long-term results.

Irritable bowel syndrome

Irritable bowel syndrome is a common disorder which is probably under diagnosed in the elderly. Although there is evidence to suggest that it is a generalized smooth muscle disorder, the aetiology and pathophysiology are not clearly defined. The Manning criteria (described later in this book) may be used to define the condition. A study of 100 individuals, aged 60–91 years, revealed abdominal pain relieved by defecation in 14 per cent and frequent straining during defecation in 20 per cent. These symptoms are often erroneously attributed to diverticular disease, which is common in this age group. Although, in younger patients, a clinical diagnosis of irritable bowel syndrome may often be made without the need for investigation, organic disease should be excluded by appropriate investigation. A recent survey from the Mayo clinic has also emphasized the frequency of functional bowel disorders in the elderly population.

Inflammatory bowel disease

Patients suffering from Crohn's colitis and ulcerative colitis survive to old age with effective treatment and careful surveillance. The two conditions may also manifest for the first time in later life. Inflammatory bowel disease in older people, though not very commonly encountered in general practice, requires careful surveillance in view of the complications associated with the condition, the effects of therapy, and the relatively poor prognosis. The prevalence of the disease varies between 10 and 70 per 100 000 population; inflammatory bowel disease is more common in whites, and approximately 40 per cent of these patients will have a family history of the disease. The disease is most common between 15 and 30 years of age, but a second peak is seen between 55 and 65 years which accounts for 10 per cent of all new cases. In an inflammatory bowel disease clinic in the University of Chicago 12 per cent of patients were at least 65 years of age and 50 per cent of these patients had developed symptoms after 50 years of age.

The natural history of the disease is similar in both old and young patients. The clinical presentation includes abdominal pain, diarrhoea, bleeding, and weight loss. Often the presentation is similar to that of diverticular disease, ischaemic bowel syndrome, and colonic malignancy. In the inflammatory bowel disease clinic in Chicago, patients who had symptoms after 50 years of age had a higher incidence of Crohn's colitis. In a Swedish study of 1655 patients with Crohn's disease the relative risk of colorectal cancer was found to be 2.5, similar to that in ulcerative colitis. In a large British series of ulcerative colitis, the cumulative probability of developing high-grade dysplasis or cancer was 4 per cent at 15 years, 7 per cent at 20 years and 13 per cent at 25 years of disease. Therefore, older patients in particular require proper assessment and appropriate surveillance. Treatment is no different from that of younger patients. Sulphasalazine is the commonly used drug for the condition although newer 5-aminosalycylic acid (5-ASA) derivatives are prescribed increasingly frequently. A low residue diet and anticholinergic drugs are used to relieve abdominal pain and diarrhoea. Some patients require iron, folic acid, and nutritional supplements because of complications of the disease or the effect of sulphasalazine on absorption of the folic acid. Some patients may require intermittent corticosteroids to control inflammation. Surgery is indicated in patients with extensive involvement of the bowel, inability to control symptoms, to deal with complications such as obstruction, perforation, bleeding, and formation of abscess and fistula. The role of prophylactic colectomy to prevent malignant change in long-standing ulcerative colitis, is controversial.

Malignant disease

The common manifestations of gastrointestinal cancer are anorexia, nausea, persistent dyspepsia, dysphagia, abdominal pain, gastrointestinal haemorrhage, diarrhoea with or without weight loss, anaemia, and fatigue. Some patients present as an emergency with obstruction or perforation.

Carcinoma of the stomach increases in incidence with age and 60 per cent of patients with the condition are over 70 years of age. The lesions are usually located in the antrum. In a large British study involving 31 000 patients, 79 per cent of them had stage IV disease and less than 1 per cent were found to have stage I gastric cancer. The high mortality, after even radical surgery, was attributed to the delay in diagnosis. The overall age-adusted five-year survival of stage IV lesions was only 5 per cent, compared with 72 per cent for those who had stage I disease. It was suggested that early detection and appropriate intervention are necessary to alter the present poor prognosis associated with the disease.

Colorectal cancer is the most common malignancy in the elderly after carcinoma of the lung in men and breast cancer in women. The peak incidence is between 75 and 85 years of age. There are 23 000 new cases of carcinoma of the colon each year and many of these diagnoses are made at a late stage. The overall five-year survival for these patients in Britain is around 15 per cent. The risk factors associated with the condition are: age greater than 50 years, a high-fat, low-fibre diet, long-standing inflammatory bowel disease, colorectal adenomas, immunodeficiency disease, and a family history of colorectal carcinoma.

It is claimed that the overall mortality of colorectal cancer can be reduced from the existing 85 per cent to 20 per cent or less if the disease is detected early. A study undertaken in Newcastle upon Tyne examined the significance of clinical findings in detecting colorectal carcinoma. Lower gastrointestinal symptoms were more common in old people with colorectal cancer, but they were also observed in healthy old people, highlighting the diagnostic difficulties in early detection of the disease. A screening study undertaken in Nottingham involved more than 100 000 people between 50 and 74 years of age. Half of the group were offered faecal occult blood testing and the other half were followed up as a control group. The initial faecal occult blood test was positive in 2.3 per cent. A total of 63 cancers and 367 adenomas were detected. The cancers detected were at a less advanced stage than those found in the control group. In an American study the predictive value of a positive Haemoccult test for colorectal cancer was reported to be 8 per cent at one year, 10 per cent at two years and 11 per cent at four years. The rates of detection were considerably higher when both adenomas and carcinomas were considered together.

Barium enema, sigmoidoscopy, and colonoscopy are the tests available to diagnose the condition once established. A retrospective review of double-contrast barium enemas in Liverpool reported weight loss, a palable mass, intestinal obstruction, positive faecal occult blood tests, and iron deficiency anaemia as important predictors of underlying bowel pathology in the elderly. Using the above criteria 93 per cent of carcinomas could be diagnosed on clinical grounds alone, although these data represent the advanced stage of disease at presentation and/or investigation.

Surgical resection is the treatment of choice. Palliative Nd:YAG laser coagulation is proving effective in managing patients with inoperable lesions. Endoscopic insertion of a Celestin tube in carcinoma of the oseophagus relieves symptoms and obstruction, which in turn permits the patients to take solid and liquid food. In patients with inoperable cancer, the main objective is to relieve pain, maintain nutrition, and provide the comfort and care the patients and their carers need.

CONCLUSION

It was not the intention of this chapter to provide a comprehensive account of all the disorders affecting the elderly gastrointestinal tract. Certain aspects of the age-specific changes in the gut and some of the commonly encountered conditions are highlighted to improve our understanding and the quality of patient care.

It is important to take an adequate history during the general practice consultation, especially if the patients have vague abdominal symptoms, weight loss, loss of appetite, change in bowel habit, unexplained anaemia, fatigue, are taking certain medication such as NSAID, and/or are suffering from other debilitating diseases. Every opportunity during the consulation should be taken to exclude serious gastrointestinal disorders, as early detection and intervention significantly alters morbidity, mortality, prognosis, and quality of life in peptic ulcer disease and in inflammatory and neoplastic conditions. Simple investigations may add ir..portant information to clinical assessment. However, in-patient hospital assessment may be more appropriate for some elderly patients, especially those who are housebound, immobile or have cognitive impairment.

FURTHER READING

Allum, W. H., Powell, D. J., McConkey, C. C., and Fielding, J. W. L. (1989). Gastric cancer: a 25 year review. *British Journal of Surgery*, **76**, 535–40.

Anderson, F. (1984). Care of the elderly: present problems and future needs. *Modern Medicine*, **29**, 11–13.

Cambell, A. J., Reinken, J., and McCosh, L. (1985). Incontinence in the elderly: prevalence and prognosis. *Age and Ageing*, **14**, 65–70.

Curless, R., French, J. M., Williams, G. and James, O. F. W. (1991). A comparison of the frequency of bowel symptoms in young and old community controls versus colorectal carcinoma patients. Presented at the British Geriatric Society Scientific Meeting, London, October 1991.

Donald, I. P., Smith, R. G., Cruikshank, J. G., Elton, R. A. and Stoddart, M. E. (1985). A study of constipation in the elderly living at home. *Gerontology*, **31**, 112–118.

Hardcastle, J. D., Thomas, W. M., Chamberlain, J. *et al.* (1989). Randomised controlled trial of faecal occult blood screening for colorectal cancer. *Lancet*, **1**, 1160–4.

Jachuck, S. (1988). Evaluation of the need in care of the elderly in a general practice. Medical Research Centre, Newcastle upon Tyne.

Talley, N. J., O'Keef, E. A., Zinsmeister, A. R., and Melton, L. J. (1992). Prevalence of gastrointestinal symptoms in the elderly: a population-based study. *Gastroenterolgy*, **102**, 895–901.

Thompson, W. G. and Heaton, K. W. (1980). Functional bowel disorders in apparently healthy people. *Gastroenterology* **79**, 283–8.

Tobin, G. W. and Brocklehurst, J. C. (1986). Faecal incontinence in residential homes for the elderly; prevalence, aetiology and management. *Age and Ageing*, **15**, 41–6.

Wald, A. (1990). Constipation and fecal incontinence in the elderly. *Gastrointestinal Clinics of North America*, **19**, 405–18.

6 Oesophageal disorders

John Galloway

The investigation and recognition of oesophageal disorders has assumed great importance in recent years, and is a major therapeutic area with significant resource implications for the National Health Service. This chapter deals with gastro-oesophageal reflux disease (GORD), motility disorders of the oesophagus, and oesophageal cancer.

STRUCTURE OF THE OESOPHAGUS

The oesophagus is a muscular tube, connecting the oropharynx to the stomach, which begins at the lower margin of the cricopharyngeus muscle and is approximately 25 cm in length. Measurements in clinical medicine are usually made with the endoscope and are expressed as the distance in centimetres from the incisor teeth. The oesophagus therefore starts at 15 cm from the incisors and ends at about 40 cm at the gastroesophageal junction. It is composed of striated muscle under voluntary control in its upper third and smooth muscle in its lower two thirds, under autonomic control from the vagus nerve. The lining mucosa is non keratinized squamous epithelium and the transformation zone to columnar epithelium is clearly seen during endoscopy (the z-line or ora serrata), marking the end of the oesophagus and beginning of the stomach. The squamous epithelium has little in the way of mucosal protective secretions to resist acid and pepsin damage from gastric juice. Just below the mucosa is a thin layer of smooth muscle, the muscularis mucosa, and deep to this is a circular and longitudinal muscle coat.

In the mediastinum the oesophagus is closely related to the two trunks of the vagus nerve, the trachea, aorta, and heart. Bronchial and aortic impressions can be seen during a barium swallow examination. A barium swallow may also show a normal mucosal pattern as three to five parallel lines of barium lying in the crenated mucosal folds. Just above the diaphragm there is an area of dilatation, known as the vestibule or phrenic ampulla, which can be confused on a barium swallow with the presence of a small hiatus hernia. The oesophagus enters the stomach at an oblique angle just below the crura of the diaphragm. Food is transported by a peristaltic wave of contraction which moves down the oesophagus at a rate of 2–6 cm/s; and if this is initiated by swallowing it is termed primary peristalsis. Secondary peristalsis originates below the hypopharynx with no antecedent swallowing.

OESOPHAGEAL FUNCTION

The *anti-reflux mechanism* is a complicated one relying on several factors. There is an area of raised intraoesophageal pressure at the lower end of the oesophagus which is designated the lower oesophageal sphincter. This high pressure zone extends 3–4 cm at the lower end of the oesophagus and can be demonstrated manometrically at levels of 15–35 mmHg. There is no anatomical sphincter in this area, so it is postulated that the raised pressure is achieved by a number of factors. These include the pinching effect around the oesophagus of the crura of the diaphragm, the acute angle between the fundus of the stomach and the entry of the oesophagus having a 'pinch cock' effect, and the arrangement of the sling fibres of the stomach which run around the angle between the oesophagus and fundus passing down the anterior and posterior walls of the stomach towards the lesser curve. These sling fibres probably work by protecting the lower oesophagus from increases in intragastric pressure by resisting distraction of the subcardiac portion of the stomach. This has been demonstrated in cadaveric stomachs and the protective effect of the sling fibres is abolished by surgical division. There is also an upper oesophageal high pressure zone which is afforded by the cricopharyngeus muscle.

Manometric studies of the normal oesophagus show that on swallowing the upper sphincter relaxes before the passage of a bolus of food, after which it contracts. This is followed by a peristaltic contraction along the oesophagus, and the lower oesophageal sphincter relaxes just before the arrival of the bolus, allowing its passage into the stomach.

The pH in the lower oesophagus is 5–7 unless there is reflux of gastric contents, which occurs briefly during swallowing. Maintenance of this pH is achieved by the anti-reflux mechanism and the continual flow of alkaline saliva (about 1500 ml/day). The clearance of acid from the lower oesophagus can be measured with intra-oesophageal pH monitoring and this technique, together with manometry, is becoming a widely used tool for assessing oesophageal function and therefore in the diagnosis of oesophageal disorders.

SYMPTOMS OF OESOPHAGEAL DISEASE

Symptoms of oesophageal disease include heartburn, odynophagia, angina-like pain, and dysphagia.

Heartburn sufferers' most common symptoms include a burning sensation in the chest (70 per cent), acid in the throat (61 per cent), flatulence and bloating (45 per cent), nausea (34 per cent), sharp chest pain (33 per cent), stomach ache (24 per cent), and difficulty in breathing (18 per cent). A working definition of heartburn is a discomfort felt moving from the low substernal or high epigastric region to the mid or high substernal region, and may be associated with regurgitation of acid or bitter tasting fluid into the mouth. Gastro-oesophageal reflux does not always produce typical heartburn and may produce cramp-like chest pain radiating to the neck, shoulder or arm, and may even be induced by emotional stress or exercise. In these latter cases, reflux may be associated with an oesophageal motor disorder. Odynophagia or pain on swallowing usually occurs in diseases which cause severe mucosal damage, such as oesophageal ulceration or severe oesophagitis. Dysphagia is associated with oesophageal obstruction, the causes of which are peptic stricture, oesophageal cancer, motility disorders including achalasia, mucosal and muscular rings, pouches and diverticulae, external compression from other mediastinal structures, and globus hystericus. Dysphagia of recent onset is a sinister symptom as it is often caused by advanced cancer.

HEARTBURN IN THE COMMUNITY

A recent Gallup poll in the UK showed that 7 per cent of the adult population use indigestion aids every day (14 per cent in Scotland) and 3 per cent of these have been doing so for more than 10 years. A total of 65 per cent of the adult population have suffered with heartburn at some point in their life and there is a slight female preponderance, presumably because of a higher incidence of heartburn in pregnancy. Heartburn occurs in all social classes with equal distribution and is a significant cause of absenteeism from work, 2 per cent of males having admitted to taking time off work due to severe symptoms and 7 per cent claiming that it interfered with their performance. It appears from the Gallup survey that heartburn has a high incidence in smokers of more than 10 cigarettes a day, heavy drinkers, and people aged 35–64 years.

INVESTIGATION OF OESOPHAGEAL DISEASE

The most common oesophageal diagnosis is GORD; this rarely causes diagnostic problems when the symptoms are typical, in which case investigations are not necessary, at least initially. Unfortunately, oesophageal pain is often difficult to distinguish from cardiac pain, especially when the conditions coexist; both may respond to sublingual glyceryl trinitrate. Usually an exercise ECG will help distinguish the two, but this should be performed under standardized conditions in hospital, where resuscitation facilities are readily available.

The investigation most commonly available to general practitioners is the barium meal, but this is by no means always helpful. It may demonstrate a hiatus hernia and reflux, but the radiologist's technique and interpretation can vary widely. Barium meals are useful for outlining strictures, benign or malignant, the presence of rings, webs, and diverticulae, and may give a clue to the presence of a motility disorder of the oesophagus. For a barium meal to show oesophagitis there must be fairly advanced linear ulceration, and the presence of a hiatus hernia is by no means always associated with oesophagitis. Many patients with a hiatus hernia never reflux. At best, barium studies serve as a screen for oesophageal disorders, but the investigation is lacking in sensitivity for the detection of reflux oesophagitis.

Gastroscopy is a better investigation, but is less available on open access. With the superb optics of the modern endoscope, minor degrees of oesophagitis can be appreciated, reflux of gastric juice into the oesophagus can be observed directly, and some assessment can be made of the integrity of the cardia, for example whether it appears lax and patulous. Strictures and rings are easily seen, and dilated during the procedure if necessary. Areas suspicious of cancer can be biopsied to add to the diagnostic accuracy. Barrett's epithelium, which is a change of normal squamous epithelium to columnar epithelium lining the oesophagus as a result of chronic gastro-oesophageal reflux, can be identified only by endoscopy and biopsy and is of importance because of its premalignant potential. A negative endoscopy however does not rule out reflux as it can occur without causing oesophagitis.

Currently the best method of assessing and diagnosing GORD is 24-hour ambulatory pH monitoring. This investigation is now becoming more widely available in district general hospital gastroenterology departments. A method gaining acceptance is the use of a pH sensitive radiotelemetry capsule which is swallowed into the oesophagus and held in place with a piece of nylon cord taped to the cheek. This 'pH capsule' measures and transmits to a recorder episodes of acid reflux over a 24-hour period and the results can be analysed from a computer printout. It would appear from the results of this investigation that reflux occurs in all individuals during the day and is associated with eating, drinking, and posture. Acid reflux episodes are cleared rapidly in normal individuals and are virtually absent during the hours of sleep. In patients with GORD, reflux episodes are more frequent and last longer and are present at night when they are supine. The enthusiasm for the test may be misplaced, as there seems to be a wide variation in the amount of reflux that occurs in normal individuals from day to day, and on some days one can get normal traces in patients who have significant reflux disease.

OESOPHAGEAL DISORDERS

Achalsia

Achalsia is caused by a defect of oesophageal motility with lack of peristalsis in the lower two thirds of the oesophagus and an incomplete relaxation of the lower oesophageal sphincter in response to voluntary swallow. It has been shown during manometric studies that the lower oesophageal sphincter is hypertensive. Cardia yield pressure, measured with a pressure transducer passed through the biopsy channel of the endoscope, is also elevated well above normal and thus a qualitative and quantitative assessment can be made of achalasia at endoscopy. This technique has also been shown to be a useful method for assessing the effectiveness of pneumatic dilatation of the cardia for this condition and formal manometry is no longer required. A barium meal will show a dilated oesophagus with lack of peristalsis and in most units remains the investigation of choice.

Diffuse oesophageal spasm

Diffuse oesophageal spasm is another motility disorder which is characterized by episodic dysphagia and chest pain resembling angina pectoris. It is not well assessed at endoscopy as the oesophagus appears normal between attacks. If at barium meal an attack of spasm occurs the tertiary contractions can be visualized—the so-called corkscrew oesophagus. More often one has to rely on oesophageal manometry which will show excessive and uncoordinated oesophageal contractions. Occasionally, diffuse oesophageal spasm is caused by oesophagitis or a distal tumour which may be better demonstrated by endoscopy.

Systemic sclerosis

Systemic sclerosis will often affect the oesophagus due to destruction of smooth muscle, leading to defective motility. Barium studies show lack of peristalsis and free reflux of gastric contents. This leads to severe oesophagitis and peptic stricture formation. Manometry will also show lack of normal peristalsis, which also may be appreciated at endoscopy, at which time it is also possible to assess the degree of mucosal damage.

Irritable bowel syndrome

No discussion of gastroenterological problems is complete without mention of irritable bowel syndrome. The condition is not confined to the small and large bowel but affects the whole of the gut. Rarely, symptoms of this condition will be confined to the area of the oesophagus, and application of the Manning criteria for clinical diagnosis of irritable bowel is unhelpful. GORD is also more common in patients with typical irritable bowel syndrome. The diagnosis may be one of exclusion after negative investigation, rather than a positive one made on the basis of clinical features.

USE OF INVESTIGATIONS

It is clear that there is no one perfect test for the diagnosis of oesophageal disorders. Reflux-related conditions and malignancy are the most common problems, so endoscopy is by far the most useful initial test for assessment and often is all that is required to make a definite diagnosis. A case is therefore made for gastroscopy to be made available on open access to all general practitioners. For this to happen more general practitioners will have to learn the technique as there are not enough gastroenterologists in the country to provide such a service; many DGH endoscopy units already rely on general practitioner endoscopists. The decision to use barium studies, manometry, and pH monitoring should be considered on the merits of the case and would perhaps be better left to a consultant gastroenterologist.

The decision to investigate early for oesophageal symptoms depends on criteria which are not strictly scientific. Patients nowadays seem generally less happy to rely on doctors' clinical assessment of their condition without a confirmatory test and the personalities of both patient and doctor will often determine the timing of investigations. Other reasons quoted in general practitioners' referral letters are the fear of missing an early and possibly treatable cancer and the need to have an accurate diagnosis before embarking on expensive forms of treatment. It is worth remembering that the cost of an endoscopy or a barium meal and a one to two month course of ranitidine (Zantac) are comparable.

Using symptoms alone as criteria for investigating upper gastrointestinal disease, the yield of positive investigations will be in the region of 20–30 per cent. A negative investigation may be very valuable on economic grounds as this may prevent the long-term use of costly drugs as well as being comforting to the patient and the doctor.

NON-CARDIAC CHEST PAIN

Of considerable current interest is the role of the oesophagus in producing chest pain of uncertain cause. This is a common problem in general practice, although precise encounter data are not available. At least 20 per cent of patients initially thought to have angina who are referred to hospital are found to have some non-cardiac cause for their pain, which is often not satisfactorily explained at all. Many more patients, who may be extremely concerned about a possible cardiac cause for their symptoms, will be dealt with by general practitioners and not referred for a specialist opinion; causes will include anxiety and hyperventilation, a variety of musculoskeletal diagnoses, and reflux-like dyspepsia. A few may have oesophagitis, biliary tract disease, and microvascular angina, which are more likely to be diagnosed on referral.

Initial explanations for the mechanisms involved in chest pain of oesophageal origin included spasm or acid sensitivity, which were reported as being responsible for as many as 60 per cent of cases of non-cardiac chest pain referred to hospital. As oesophageal studies—pH monitoring and pressure studies—have become more widely available, so a whole family of oesophageal disorders, thought to cause non-cardiac chest pain, has been described. The conditions most commonly identified include nutcracker oesophagus, where there are peristaltic waves of excessive amplitude, diffuse oesophageal spasm in which frequent simultaneous non-peristaltic contractions occur, hypertensive lower oesophageal sphincter, and non-specific motility disorder. The prevalence of these conditions and, indeed, the criteria for their diagnosis vary considerably between research centres, and recent reviews have pointed out that rather than representing a 'new' explanation for non-cardiac chest pain, these disorders are in fact uncommon in unselected patients in the community and in primary care. For example,the manometric events which are said to characterize nutcracker oesophagus and diffuse spasm may occur in normal subjects and are accentuated by stress. Psychiatric diagnoses are made significantly more frequently in patients with oesophageal motor dysfunction than in those without, and patients who complain of 'oesophageal' chest pain have a lower general pain threshold than normal controls. Antidepressant treatment has been shown to relieve the pain without changing the dysmotility patterns.

The question for the general practitioner is what to do in patients with chest pain in whom ischaemic heart disease and oesophagitis have been excluded. A therapeutic trial of acid suppression may be a quicker and cheaper alternative to referral for pH monitoring. Pressure studies may demonstrate a motility disorder, but therapy is not always straightforward or successful, although a positive diagnosis may help in mangement. Given the good general prognosis for patients with disorders of this kind, explanation and reassurance analogous to that provided in irritable bowel syndrome may be the most appropriate management for most patients, with referral and oesophageal studies being reserved for those in whom these simple measures fail.

MANAGEMENT OF GORD

Although non-drug management and life-style advice are fundamental in treating GORD, it is also important to understand the role of drug therapy in management.

Role of drugs in reflux disease

Antacids

These neutralize gastric acid to a certain extent, and therefore reduce the acid insult to the oesophageal mucosa during reflux. They also increase lower oesophageal sphincter pressure and reduce reflux. Despite these proven effects there is no good clinical trial evidence that antacids are superior to placebo. In clinical practice, nevertheless, antacids do appear to be effective in the control of mild to moderate symptoms of reflux. Gaviscon is a popular antacid use for reflux symptoms and contains a mixture of sodium bicarbonate, calcium carbonate, and sodium alginate (available as liquid or tablets—dosage 10–20 ml or 2 tablets after meals and at night). The mode of action is said to be that the alginate produces a raft of neutral pH which impedes reflux, and the alkalis neutralize gastric acid. When reflux occurs the raft protects the oesophageal mucosa from direct acid injury. There have been numerous trials on the efficiency of alginic acid in reflux disease and few suggest any real benefit over simple antacids. The relatively high sodium content of Gaviscon (6.2 mmol per 10 ml) may be a disadvantage in patients suffering with congestive heart failure or renal failure. The long-term use of aluminium-containing antacids should probably be avoided in view of the association between Alzheimer's disease and aluminium ingestion, although there are no data comparing tissue levels of long-term antacid users with controls and the main problem appears to be in patients suffering with renal failure on dialysis.

Bethanechol

Bethanechol (Myotonine) is a cholinergic agent which causes an increase in lower oesophageal sphincter pressure and acid clearance from the lower oesophagus and can be used separately or in combination with other drugs (dosage 10–30 mg, 3–4 times a day, half an hour before food). It is more popular in the USA than in the UK.

Metoclopramide and domperidone

Metoclopramide (Maxolon, Primperan, 10 mg three times a day before food) and domperidone (Motilium, Evoxin, 10 mg three times a day before food) are dopamine antagonists which increase lower oesophageal sphincter pressure and gastric emptying, but there is no evidence that either increase acid clearance from the oesophagus. Trials have shown a significant improvement in symptoms and decrease in antacid consumption with these drugs. Metoclopramide crosses the blood–brain barrier more effectively than domperidone and has a higher incidence of central nervous system side-effects, including restlessness, insomnia, anxiety, and extrapyramidal reactions, especially in children and in the elderly. Combination of metoclopramide with cimetidine shows no significant difference compared with cimetidine alone in healing oesophagitis and reduction of symptoms. The combination may produce more side-effects, because of cimetidine's effect on the hepatic metabolism of other drugs.

Cisapride

Cisapride (Prepulsid, 10 mg three times a day) is a newly developed compound that increases gastrointestinal motility by increasing the release of acetylcholine from the mysenteric plexus. It increases the basal lower oesophageal sphincter pressure in fasting healthy subjects. It has no anti-dopaminergic side-effects like domperidone and metoclopramide and is being marketed as a useful drug in the treatment of gastro-oesophageal reflux. It is only possible to give an interim opinion on its place for treatment of GORD. So far it appears to be as good as H_2-antagonists for treating GORD and may be cheaper than using these drugs in high dosage. It does not have the central nervous system side-effects of metaclopramide, but can cause diarrhoea and abdominal cramps. It also shows considerable promise as an agent for maintenance treatment in GORD patients, and several studies have shown that adding cisapride to cimetidine results in significantly more healing and symptom relief than the H_2-antagonist alone. The recommended dose of cisapride is 10 mg three or four times daily. The drug has a long half-life and thus this frequency would seem unnecessary, twice a day being more logical and of course a cheaper option. The dose should be halved for patients with renal or hepatic failure and in the elderly, and the drug should not be used in pregnancy or in lactating mothers.

Histamine-2-receptor antagonists

Histamine-2-receptor antagonists (cimetidine, 800 mg twice daily, ranitidine, 300 mg twice daily) act by reducing gastric acid production and, in the majority of trials, have been shown to lead to significant symptom improvement and a decrease in antacid consumption. The doses needed seem to be double that required for duodenal ulcer healing and the effect on oesophagitis healing rate is much less reliable. The effect on reduction of peptic strictures is disappointing. Patients with endoscopically proven oesophagitis require long-term H$_2$-antagonists rather than the short courses used in duodenal ulcer. There is no difference in the efficiency of ranitidine over cimetidine in the treatment of GORD and the side-effects of cimetidine are barely different to those of ranitidine. The problems of drug interaction with cimetidine are overstated and easily overcome by checking blood levels in the case of theophylline preparations, and prothrombin time in the case of warfarin. If cimetidine was the only H$_2$-antagonist available in the UK the saving to the heath service has been estimated to be in the region of £17 million, this representing the difference in cost incurred by the prescription of ranitidine. This is very relevant in the climate of reducing drug spending.

Sucralfate

Sucralfate (Antepsin, 2 g twice daily) binds specifically to ulcerated lesions, bile, and acid and therefore may be useful in improving the mucosal barier to acid, pepsin, and bile attack.

Omeprazole

Omeprazole (Losec, 20–40 mg once daily) to date is the most effective drug for healing all forms of peptic ulceration in the upper gastrointestinal tract. It is a substituted benzimidazole which inhibits the K$^+$/H$^+$ transporting ATPase in the parietal cells and thereby results in almost complete supression of basal and stimulated acid secretion. The results of omeprazole are so far impressive, with a dose of 20–40 mg per day for 4–8 weeks resulting in remarkable symptomatic and endoscopic improvement. There are two theoretical problems with the use of this drug. The first is that rendering the stomach achlorhydric removes a valuable defence against

Table 6.1 *Summary of drug trial results in GORD*

Drug	Symptomatic improvement	Oesophagitis healing	Healing of strictures
Antacids	?	?	Unknown
Alginic acid	Yes	?	Unknown
Bethanechol	Yes	Yes	Unknown
Metoclopramide	Yes	?	Unknown
Cisapride	Yes	Yes	Unknown
H$_2$-antagonists	Yes	Yes	No
Omeprazole	Yes	Yes	Yes

gut-borne infections, and the second is that prolonged use results in hypergastrinaemia and enterochromaffin-like-cell proliferation in the stomach, which may be a precursor to gastric carcinoid. These problems however, are theoretical and omeprazole is now licensed for long-term use in GORD.

The results of trials of drug treatments in reflux are summarized in Table 6.1.

STAGES OF TREATMENT OF GORD

The majority of patients with GORD should be managed by their general practitioner. Patients with chronic reflux symptoms should be investigated before the long-term use of relatively expensive drugs is contemplated.

Before one can treat reflux successfully an understanding of the pathophysiology of the condition is required. Until relatively recently investigators concentrated most of their work on the lower oesophageal sphincter mechanisms, considering that failure of this was crucial in the development of reflux disease. Because an anatomical sphincter does not exist, most workers now accept that the anti-reflux barrier is created by a combination of factors working at the lower end of the oesophagus and upper part of the stomach. Treatment aims at combating the following factors which are defective in gastroesophageal reflux:

(1) the efficiency of the anti-reflux barrier at the oesophago-gastric junction;
(2) the irritant effect of gastric juice (acid, pepsin, and bile);
(3) the efficiency of the oesophageal clearing mechanism (peristalsis, salivary flow, and bicarbonate);
(4) oesophageal mucosal barrier to acid digestion;
(5) efficiency of gastric emptying.

With these factors in mind initial treatment should be in the form of advice to patients about life-style.

Stage 1

Stop smoking

Smoking causes a marked lowering of LES (lower oesophageal sphincter) pressure: two cigarettes over a 20-minute period can result in a 50 per cent reduction. The mechanism of action is probably that of nicotine blocking the cholinergic control of the LES. Intraoesophageal pH studies have shown a significant association between reflux and smoking.

Blocking up the head end of the bed

Again, pH studies have shown that reflux sufferers have prolonged acid explosure to the oesophagus when supine. Blocking the head of the bed and raising it by 15–20 cm will assist oesophageal clearance of acid by gravity and has substantial effects on diminishing symptoms and healing oesophagitis.

Dietary modification

Certain foods lower LES pressure and delay gastric emptying increasing reflux; these include fats, alcohol, and carminatives (peppermint) which are best avoided in reflux sufferers. Foods which have a direct irritant effect on the oesophageal mucosa, for example, citrus fruit, tomatoes, and coffee should be avoided. Coffee has the added disadvantage of stimulating gastric acid secretion and decreasing LES pressure. Conversely, foods rich in protein increase LES pressure and therefore reduce reflux.

Weight loss

Losing weight is a traditional component of reflux treatment and loss of a few crucial pounds may help symptoms, but there is no trial evidence to support this. It is more likely that dietary modification used to achieve weight loss is responsible for improvement in symptoms.

In addition to this advice the reflux sufferer should be prescribed a simple antacid for symptomatic relief of heartburn. There is no evidence that expensive antacids containing alginate are superior.

The next stage in management of oesophageal pain will involve the use of other drugs, preferably after appropriate investigation.

Stage 2

If the symptoms persist despite judicious changes in life-style, as outlined above, providing the patient is under the age of 45 years a course of an H_2-antagonist with or without metoclopramide can be tried for six weeks. If this does not settle the symptoms, or if the symptoms recur after cessation of treatment, the patient should be investigated. Earlier investigation is indicated if there is a history of dysphagia, vomiting, odynophagia, and angina-like chest pain associated with reflux in the patient over the age of 45 years presenting for the first time with reflux symptoms. If investigations are contemplated then it is wise to stop H_2-antagonists at least two weeks beforehand, as the healing properties of these drugs may mask the true severity of the oesophagitis. At present omeprazole is not recommended for use as 'blind' symptomatic therapy, but is increasingly used as a first-line treatment in GORD.

Investigation should proceed with endoscopy or barium studies according to local facilities and move on to pH monitoring and/or manometry if there is diagnostic difficulty as outlined above.

Treatment of oesophagitis should be with long-term H_2-antagonists or omeprazole with or without metoclopramide, domperidone or cisapride. Pain produced by osesophageal spasm confirmed by manometry can be helped by smooth muscle relaxants, such as the calcium channel blocker, nifedipine 10 mg, taken before food. The liquid in nifedipine capsules can be absorbed buccally for a faster onset of action.

In the event of failure of this stage of treatment or patient unacceptability, management tends to move from the realm of general practice and the question of anti-reflux surgery needs to be considered with the guidance of a consultant gastroenterologist.

The indications for anti-reflux surgery are listed below.

Stage 3

Severe oesophagitis with peptic stricture and/or Barrett's mucosal changes in the oesophagus is difficult to manage without specialist advice. Barrett's oesophagus was first described in 1950 as a circumferential involvement of at least the lowermost 3 cm of the oesophagus with columnar epithelium as a consequence of chronic reflux. Columnar epithelium is found in 10–16 per cent of patients with chronic reflux. The prevalence of adenocarcinoma in columnar-epithelium is 8–15 per cent.

A postal follow-up of 155 patients with columnar epithelium concluded that endoscopic surveillance is not indicated. In this retrospective study of patients with columnar epithelium diagnosed over a 12-year period the incidence of oesophageal carcinoma was 1 in 170 patient years, representing a 30-fold increase in risk over the general population. The survival of patients with Barrett's oesophagus was not different from an age and sex matched population. Barrett's changes do therefore carry a risk of the development of adenocarcinoma, but the risk is overstated. Those patients most as risk have greater than 8 cm of altered mucosa extending up the oesophagus, with dysplasia in that mucosa, and the presence of intestinal metaplasia, which is a histological change often seen in the mucosa surrounding an oesophageal adenocarcinoma. Some gastroenterologists examine all patients with Barrett's oesophagus on a yearly basis. This is clearly a waste of resources, and should be reserved for patients with the above changes. It remains to be seen whether long-term treatment with omeprazole leads to regression of the columnar mucosa.

In patients with severe forms of oesophagitis, surgery should be contemplated, especially if they are young or if the reflux is causing micro-aspiration of gastric contents. Such chronic aspiration can lead to asthma due to increased bronchial reactivity, pneumonia, and basal fibrosis. These conditions are more commonly associated with achalasia and scleroderma, but chronic pulmonary disease secondary to GORD is probably under diagnosed. The effects of long-term H_2-antagonist or omeprazole therapy are unknown and patients suffering with the more severe types of the condition will not spontaneously improve. Anti-reflux surgery has a 90 per cent success rate and involves procedures to strengthen the anti-reflux mechanism. The most widely used procedures are the Nissen and Belsey fundoplication, which involve the wrapping of the fundus of the stomach around the lower oesophagus.

In patients who are not candidates for surgery because of age or the presence of precluding illness, the use of intermittent courses of omeprazole interpersed with H_2-antagonists and domperidone or metoclopramide is the best alternative. Periodic endoscopy may be needed to monitor the success of this regime, as symptoms are not reliable in assessing the healing of oesophagitis.

1. Failure of medical treatment, patient compliance.
2. Recurrent peptic stricture formation.
3. Development of aspiration-induced pulmonary disease.
4. More severe forms of Barrett's oesophagus.

FOLLOW-UP MEDICAL TREATMENT

1. Patients who are initially treated on stage 1 of the management protocol should be reviewed at one month, and if the doctor and patient are happy with symptom control then no follow-up is required.
2. If initiated on stage 2 treatment, review should be at 6 weeks initially. Ideally thereafter at 3-monthly intervals if on long-terms H_2-antagonists or omeprazole to check on symptom control and the development of new symptoms, such as dysphagia and respiratory problems. Any new symptoms should be referred for further endoscopic assessment.
3. Patients with severe oesophagitis receiving courses of omeprazole should be under review by a gastroenterologist as well as their general practitioner. Selected cases with Barrett's changes in the oesophagus should be reviewed endoscopically in view of their malignant potential.

In conclusion, many patients with proven oesophagitis will be dependent on long-term if not life-long therapy to control their symptoms. As the main cause of the problem in these cases is an incompetent anti-reflux mechanism, surgery may be the best choice in properly selected patients.

The stages of treatment of gastro-oesophageal reflux are listed below.

Stage 1
(a) Modify diet;
(b) Stop smoking;

(c)   Simple antacids;
(d)   Elevate head of bed;
(e)   Avoid drugs which can cause peptic ulceration.

Stage 2
(a)   H$_2$-antagonists, intermittent omeprazole;
(b)   Metoclopramide/domperidone/cisapride;
(c)   ? Sucralfate;
(d)   + stage 1.

Stage 3
(a)   Long-term omeprazole;
(b)   Referral;
(c)   Anti-reflux surgery.

MOTILITY DISORDERS OF THE OESOPHAGUS

The diagnosis of these disorders has been dealt with above. Motility disorders can be classified as primary or secondary. Primary disorders include achalasia and diffuse oesophageal spasm, while secondary motility disorders occur in scleroderma, other connective tissue disorders, diabetes mellitus, Chagas disease, muscle disorders, such as dystrophia myotonica, neurological disorders, such as multiple sclerosis and motor neurone disease, and finally as part of the ageing process—presbyoesophagus.

The treatment of secondary motility disorders is different from that of achalasia and diffuse oesophageal spasm, in that no drug can be used to restore either lost smooth muscle or reverse denervation and the problem is one of an atonic oesophagus allowing reflux and its consequences, including oesophagitis, stricture formation, and aspiration of gastric contents leading to chronic respiratory disorders. The use of H$_2$-antagonists, omeprazole, and prokinetic agents all have their place, and stricture dilatation will be required in selected patients. Anti-reflux surgery may be required in some patients, especially if there is aspiration of gastric contents, but great skill is required to ensure that anti-reflux operations are not too tight at the cardia, as severe dysphagia will ensue.

Achalasia

A smooth muscle relaxant, preferably nifedepine 10–20 mg taken sublingually immediately before meals or whenever symptoms occur, may be used to treat early cases of achalasia without significant oesophageal dilatation. Once the oesophagus is dilated and the patient is suffering with dysphagia and regurgitation pneumatic dilatation is required. The object of the exercise is to reduce the yield pressure of the cardia as measured through the endoscope to near zero. If this is achieved then more dilatation will not improve symptoms further. In difficult cases longitudinal oeso-phagomyotomy will be required in order to achieve this low yield pressure but these cases are very infrequent. After successful dilatation reflux once more becomes a problem.

Diffuse oesophageal spasm and hypercontractile oesophagus

Patients with this condition are advised to avoid all types of food and drink that have aggravated the symptoms in the past. In addition, nifedepine 10–20 mg before meals may be useful. Some patients respond better to nitrates, such as glyceryl trinitrate sublingually before meals or hydralazine 25–75 mg three times a day. In refractory cases pneumatic dilatation or even oesophagomyotomy may be considered.

Oesophageal cancer

The predominant presenting symptom of oesophageal cancer is dysphagia, by which time approximately two-thirds of the oesophageal lumen is involved.

About 70 per cent of patients have inoperable lesions at diagnosis and five-year survival after radical surgery is less than 5 per cent. The mortality following oesophagectomy is about 29 per cent. It is not surprising, therefore, that in the majority of cases palliation is all that can be offered.

Carcinoma of the oesophagus is classified according to site and cell type (squamous cell or adenocarcinoma). Tumours of the upper third of the oesophagus comprise about 20 per cent and are predominantly squamous lesions. They are usually radiosensitive and because of the magnitude of surgical excision involving a pharyngo-laryngectomy, radiotherapy is the treament of choice. Tumours of the lower two thirds occur with equal frequency. The majority of middle third lesions are squamous, although adenocarcinomata can occur in islands of gastric epithelium and from mucus glands and columnar lined oesophagus (Barrett's osophagus) which results from chronic long-term reflux. The majority of lower third tumours are adenocarcinomas and are really gastric cancers which have migrated upwards.

The treatment options for oesophageal cancer are surgery, therapeutic endoscopy, radiotherapy, and chemotherapy. The object of treatment is to offer a cure in a few cases and to improve swallowing and hopefully avoid an unpleasant death due to starvation. Careful assessment of the patients is therefore required with factors such as age of patient, cell type, and evidence of spread taken into account before any treatment is undertaken. In the large majority of cases the endoscopic placement of an Atkinson tube is the least invasive and offers the best survival rates with least morbidity. The details and controversies of these treatments are discussed in Chapter 12.

The best hope of managing this condition is prevention and at present the associated factors seem to be chronic reflux and smoking. Following selected patients with Barrett's oesophagus with regular endoscopy and active treatment to reduce exposure of the oesophagus to acid reflux may help to reduce the incidence of this condition. Encouraging patients to stop smoking is vital in the prevention of this and many other conditions.

FURTHER READING

Atkinson, M. (1989). Barrett's oesophagus—to screen or not to screen. *Gut*, **30**, 2–4.

Bardhan, K. D., Morris, P., Thompson, M., Dhande, D. S., Hinchcliffe, R. F., Jones, R. B. *et al.* (1990). Omeprazole in the treatment of erosive oesophagitis refectory to high dose cimetidine and ranitidine. *Gut*, **31**, 745–9.

Brown, S. G. (1991). Palliation of malignant dysphagia: surgery, radiotherapy, laser intubation alone or in combination? *Gut*, **32**, 841–4.

Colin-Jones, D. G. (1989). Histamine-2-receptor antagonists in gastro-oesophageal reflux. *Gut*, **30**, 1305–8.

Dehn, T. C. B. (1992). Surgery for uncomplicated gastro-oesophageal reflux. *Gut*, **33**, 293–4.

DeMeester, T. R., Bonavina, L. and Albertucci, M. (1986). Nissen fundoplication for gastro-oesophageal reflux disease. *Annals of Surgery*, **204**, 9–20.

Lancet (Editorial) (1991). The oesophagus and chest pain of uncertain cause. *Lancet*, **339**, 583–4.

McGouran, R. C. M., Galloway, J. M., Spence, D. S., Morton, C. P. and Marchant, D. (1988). Does measurement of yield pressure at the cardia during endoscopy provide information on the function of the lower oesophageal sphincter mechanism? *Gut*, **29**, 275–8.

Toussaint, J., Gossuin, A., Deruyttere, M., Huble, F. and Devis, G. (1991). Healing and prevention of relapse of reflux oesophagitis by cisapride. *Gut*, **32**, 1280–5.

Valori, R. M. (1990). Nutcracker, neurosis or sampling bias? *Gut*, **31**, 736–7.

Watson, A. and Atkinson, M. (1991). Provision of facilities for manometry and pH monitoring in the investigation of patients with oesophageal disease. *Gut*, **32**, 106–7.

7 Peptic ulceration

Robert Walt and Roger Jones

From a number of perspectives, peptic ulcer disease is the most important organic gastroenterological condition. It affects, at some time, approximately 10 per cent of all adults males in the West. In general practice in the UK the annual incidence of new cases of peptic ulcer is at least 5 per 1000 registered patients each year, with at least 100 people on each general practitioner's list having had a diagnosis of peptic ulcer at some time. In terms of morbidity and mortality, peptic ulcer should not be underestimated. Dyspeptic symptoms and ulceration itself represent significant causes of time lost from work and lost productivity, as well as social security costs. Figures for the UK are difficult to obtain, but the economic cost of peptic ulceration in the USA is said to be around $1 billion each year. Peptic ulcer-related deaths number about 4500 each year in the UK; 30 000 people are admitted with upper gastrointestinal haemorrhage alone, and 10 per cent of them die. The prescribing costs related to peptic ulceration are also considerable. Effective acid-suppressing agents have been available for many years and account for about half of all prescriptions written for gastrointestinal drugs. At present, each general practitioner's prescribing costs for gastrointestinal drugs are around £10 000 per year.

The investigation of patients suspected of having peptic ulceration or developing complications also has enormous resource consequences, particularly in terms of the increasingly sophisticated diagnostic and therapeutic technology which has developed, including fibre-optics, video-endoscopy, and lasers.

EPIDEMIOLOGY

The prevalence and pattern of peptic ulcer disease and symptoms of dyspepsia in the community and in the hospital setting have changed substantially during recent decades. However, studies performed at different times may be difficult to compare because of different methods of ascertainment used in each. For example, in 1951 the influence of occupational factors in the aetiology of gastric and duodenal ulcers was investigated in more than 6000 employees working for a number of companies in London. They were asked whether they had ever had a peptic ulcer or had suffered from indigestion. On the basis of interviews conducted by a social worker, the subjects were classified into either major dyspepsia, minor dyspepsia (people with indigestion who had not vomited blood, been diagnosed as having a peptic ulcer, had a barium meal, or whose symptoms were not 'suggestive' of peptic ulcer in the last five years), or no dyspepsia. More than 1000 (17 per cent) of the subjects had minor dyspepsia, and that 819 (13 per cent) had major dyspepsia; those with major dyspepsia were interviewed and 334 peptic ulcers were diagnosed, of which 69 per cent were presumptive diagnoses based on history alone. The general conclusions of this study were that almost 30 per cent of the sample had suffered dyspepsia in the last five years and that almost 2 per cent had peptic ulcers. Clearly, estimates of this kind, in which the clinical history alone is used as a diagnostic criterion cannot be compared with endoscopically-controlled studies performed more recently.

One interesting starting point is the observation, confirmed in a number of studies in recent years, that the point prevalence of active duodenal ulceration in apparently normal, healthy people is at least 1 per cent. The natural history of these 'unreported' ulcers is not known with certainty, but it seems likely that the majority of them run a benign, possibly entirely self-limiting course. This observation makes it rather difficult to be sure about the significance of ulcers as a cause for symptoms in every case, and about the natural history of ulcers diagnosed at endoscopy on the basis of 'typical' symptoms. Additionally, the placebo healing rate of ulcers in most clinical trials approaches 30–40 per cent, suggesting that even 'significant' ulcers frequently run a benign course. It is important to recognize a spectrum of severity and significance in duodenal ulcer disease, ranging from almost incidentally-discovered lesions to severe ulceration producing complications and leading to significant morbidity and mortality.

Current best estimates are that the lifetime prevalence of peptic ulceration for men is about 10 per cent, with women having a lifetime prevalence of about half that. These figures are supported by a large autopsy study of 13 000 patients performed in Leeds, when chronic duodenal ulcer was found in 7.8 per cent of men and 4 per cent of women who had died from causes other than peptic ulcer. The data in this study suggested that, over the age of 35 years, at least 13 per cent of men and 5 per cent of women suffer from duodenal ulcer and 3.9 per cent of men from gastric ulcer. In a further study in north-east Scotland, when a near-static population of men was investigated, 8 per cent of those aged 15–64 years were found to have peptic ulcers. The point prevalence of active peptic ulcer disease is probably in the range of 1–2 per cent.

Incidence rates of duodenal ulcer are thought to be about 0.18 per cent per year in men and women together. The age-specific incidence increases almost linearly with age, reaching 0.3 per cent in men in their late 70s. Gastric ulcers are generally less frequent than duodenal ulcers; about 80 per cent of all peptic ulcers are situated in the duodenum. The annual incidence figure for gastric ulcers in men and women is of the order of 0.03 per cent. However, in terms of complications, the distribution is more even. In the most recent studies of peptic ulcer bleeding the frequency of gastric and duodenal ulcer as causes for the bleeding was more or less equal.

Duodenal ulcer was, curiously, infrequently recognized before the beginning of this century and its occurrence increased steadily until about 1960. A number of indirect indicators can be used to measure the incidence of duodenal ulcer disease, including rates of hospitalization, operation, and death, and all of these suggest a marked decrease in duodenal ulcer incidence in England, Europe, and the USA in the last 20–30 years. There has been a decline in hospital admissions for duodenal ulcer in England and Wales, although hospitalization rates for duodenal ulcer disease complicated by haemorrhage or perforation have not changed so much. Admissions for gastric ulcer and unspecified peptic ulcer have also increased, possibly because of an increase in the proportion of these ulcers complicated by haemorrhage. In addition to these changes, there has been an increase in perforation and death rates from duodenal ulcer in women aged 60 years and over, paralleling an increase in the prescription of NSAIDs to this group of patients. The prescription rate of these drugs has risen dramatically in the last 20 years, with more than 25 million prescriptions now being issued annually. In addition, there has been a change over the last 30–40 years in the sex ratio of patients with chronic duodenal ulcer disease. In the 1930s the ratio of men to women was about 4.5:1, rising to a peak of 4.7:1 in the mid 1940s, and falling to 2:1 in the 1960s. The reason for this is not clear.

Efforts to elucidate the aetiology of peptic ulcer disease have frequently involved epidemiological studies in other cultures, particularly in developing countries. Studies in Africa and India, for example, show a high incidence of duodenal ulcer disease in some rural areas, characterized by a high ratio of duodenal to gastric ulcer, a high male to female ratio, a peak age incidence 10 years earlier than in Western societies, and a high incidence of pyloric stenosis. These observations are at odds with the stereotypical association between peptic ulcer disease and a stressed executive life-style. Although the original survey in London reported that the incidence of duodenal ulcer was greater in men holding 'responsible positions' and that 'anxiety over work or personality factors leading to anxiety' were unduly common in subjects with duodenal ulcer, duodenal ulcer now occurs uniformly in all social groups. In this study the frequency of gastric ulceration was related to social and economic class, being least frequent in the wealthiest classes and most frequent in the poorest and in unskilled and manual workers. In a recent Scandinavian survey of peptic ulcer disease, an equal sex ratio was noted, half of all new peptic ulcers occurred in people over the age of 60 years and 20 per cent of all ulcer diagnoses were made in patients presenting with gastrointestinal haemorrhage, confirming trends previously reported in the UK and USA.

NATURAL HISTORY

Peptic ulcer is a chronic recurrent disease, with the majority of patients suffering a relapse within a year of initial diagnosis. In duodenal ulcer, the onset is usually between the age of 20 and 40 years, and symptoms tend to recur periodically for at least 5–10 years, although in a substantial number of patients a spontaneous gradual reduction in recurrence rate occurs, and some may eventually enter a period of prolonged remission. In a long-term follow-up of duodenal ulcer, in general practice, disease symptoms finally ceased altogether in later life in many patients. This course of onset, peak, spontaneous remission, and recovery occurred in about 60 per cent of patients with duodenal ulcer. However, asymptomatic ulcers are not uncommon in elderly people, so absence of symptoms can not be equated with cure. In another 29 per cent, however, the symptoms were severe and persistent, requiring surgical intervention, although it must be remembered that these figures were, in part, derived before the use of potent ulcer-healing agents was widespread. In the same series, 20 per cent of patients were said to develop the complications of bleeding and perforation.

The peak age of onset of gastric ulcer tends to be later, between 50 and 70 years of age, with a clinical course similar to that seen in duodenal ulcer and a distinct tendency towards spontaneous recovery. In this series, surgery was required in 25 per cent of gastric ulcers, bleeding occurred in 10 per cent, and perforation in less than 1 per cent.

Other studies have also questioned the assertion 'once an ulcer, always an ulcer'. For example, in one group of patients followed for 13 years in the USA, 68 per cent had become asymptomatic or had only mild symptoms, with only 12 per cent having moderate to severe symptoms and 20 per cent having had surgery for duodenal ulcer. These are very similar figures to early observations made in British general practice, although cases diagnosed in general practice seem to follow a milder course than those diagnosed in a hospital setting, so that the groups may not be strictly comparable. Depending on the population under study, therefore, perhaps two thirds of duodenal ulcer patients may experience symptom 'burn out' over a period of 10–15 years. The results of long-term trials of maintenance therapy to prevent recurrence have also indicated that recurrences tend to be more frequent during the early years of the trials, with lower rates occurring during subsequent years. However, an alternative explanation for these observations is that patients with the most severe ulcers relapse early and leave the study.

For practical purposes, however, duodenal ulcer disease should be regarded as a life-long chronic condition with implications for follow-up and surveillance similar to those for other chronic disorders.

Finally, the lifetime risk of serious complications of duodenal ulcers could be as high as 20 per cent, assuming that ulcer disease is active for a period of 8–15 years; perhaps 1–3 per cent of patients with duodenal ulcer develop complications during the course of each year of disease. In terms of mortality, actuarial analysis indicates that life expectancy for patients with duodenal ulcer is only modestly decreased, and this during the first year or two after diagnosis, with little change in life expectancy in later years. Patients with both duodenal and gastric ulcers have a rather higher mortality rate, but the benign nature of duodenal ulcer disease in general practice is well demonstrated by the occurrence in Fry's 15-year follow-up of 265 patients of only one duodenal ulcer related death.

CAUSES OF PEPTIC ULCERATION

Although Schwartz's dictum 'no acid, no ulcer' implicates gastric acid as a central causative factor in peptic ulcer disease, in reality the development of an ulcer is almost certainly the result of the interaction of several factors, with the relative importance of these varying in different individuals and in different forms of ulceration. Duodenal ulcers represent a break in the mucosa of the duodenum extending through the muscularis mucosae, with an ulcer crater surrounded by acute and chronic inflammatory cell infiltrate. The ulcer is usually situated in the first part of the duodenum, just distal to the junction of pyloric and duodenal mucosa; occasionally it may be distal to this and is called a postbulbar ulcer. Half of these ulcers are on the anterior wall of the duodenum, 23 per cent on the posterior wall. About 10–15 per cent of duodenal ulcers are multiple.

Benign gastric ulcer is a non-neoplastic localized break in mucosal continuity extending through the muscularis mucosae of the stomach wall. The ulcers usually occur at or near the mucosal transitional junctions on the lesser curvature of the stomach and the prepyloric antrum.

GASTRIC SECRETION

Secretion of both acid and pepsin appears to be necessary for the development of peptic ulcers; duodenal ulcers do not develop when there is achlorhydria, but invariably occur in the Zollinger–Ellison syndrome, in which there is hypersecretion of gastric acid. The role of acid is, however, far from clear. Whilst, as a group, patients with duodenal ulcer secrete more acid, both basally and in response to a variety of stimuli, than normal subjects, the majority of them have acid secretion profiles falling within a statistically defined normal range, such as the mean plus or minus two standard deviations.

Other observations have been made which lend more support to the role of acid in causing peptic ulceration. In prospective studies on ulcer-free subjects, for example those with higher acid outputs were more likely to develop ulcers during follow-up. Patients with duodenal ulcer seemed to have a lower intra-duodenal pH for longer periods than control subjects, both fasting and in response to food. Other data suggest that the acid response to food is greater and more prolonged in duodenal ulcer subjects than in normal subjects. There may be excessive drive to acid secretion, with blood gastrin levels in duodenal ulcer subjects higher after a meal than in controls. As well as increased numbers or hyperplasia of parietal cells, there may be increased sensitivity of these acid-secreting cells, and possibly impaired inhibitory mechanisms for acid secretion.

MUCOSAL RESISTANCE

While acid and pepsin can be regarded as aggressive factors, which tend to attack the mucosae of the stomach and duodenum, a number of protective mechanisms exist to prevent mucosal damage. These include an ionic 'mucosal barrier', effective cell repair and renewal, mucus and mucosal bicarbonate secretion, and adequate mucosal blood flow, related, probably, to local synthesis of prostaglandins. Gastric mucus plays an important role by trapping bicarbonate ions within its interstices, permitting neutralization of hydrogen ions. The integrity of the mucosal epithelium depends on tight junctions between cells and the surface lipoprotein layer of the epithelial cells, which can all be damaged by ulcer-inducing agents, such as aspirin and NSAIDs. Bicarbonate secretion is itself stimulated by prostaglandins synthesized in the gastric mucosa; inhibition of prostaglandin synthesis will not only decrease bicarbonate secretion, but will also have adverse local effects on the micro-circulation of the mucosa. Many of these prostaglandins are regarded as 'cytoprotective' because of their role in the prevention of damage from noxious agents.

The simplistic view of the pathogenesis of peptic ulceration is to consider the balance between these aggressive and protective factors, with ulceration occurring when inadequate defence mechanisms are breached by normal or excessive 'attack' factors, principally acid and pepsin, but also including a variety of drugs, such as NSAIDs.

HELICOBACTER PYLORI

The 'acid story' has been upset for some years since evidence has accumulated about the association between gastric colonization with the organism *Helicobacter pylori* and duodenal ulceration. These curved bacilli were first described in the gastric mucosa in 1983 and intense interest now centres around the relationship between them, non-autoimmune gastritis, and peptic ulceration. The organism is a Gram-negative rod, which often appears bent or spiral, and is sensitive to a variety of antibiotics and bismuth compounds.

There seems little doubt that *H. pylori* is associated with the development of non-autoimmune gastritis and there is increasing evidence for a causative rather than coincidental role in duodenal ulcer disease. This conclusion is based on the finding that almost all patients with active duodenal ulceration can be shown, using a variety of diagnostic tests, to be *Helicobacter*-positive. The percentage positivity rate rises with age and is roughly equal to the patient's age in years, so that colonization is observed in normal subjects, but is almost invariable in patients with duodenal ulcer disease, so much so that a recent international working party determined that in patients with endoscopically-proven duodenal ulcer disease biopsy or other testing for *Helicobacter* was pointless.

In addition to this strong association, eradication of *H. pylori* by administering bismuth in conjunction with one or more antibiotics is linked to a much lower relapse rate for duodenal ulcer disease than is observed in patients treated with acid-suppressing drugs only. In the year following a single therapeutic course of an H_2-receptor antagonist, 70–80 per cent of duodenal ulcers will relapse, unless maintenance treatment is given. Following a therapeutic course of, for example, colloidal bismuth subcitrate in conjunction with amoxycillin and metronidazole, the annual relapse rate can be shown to fall to around 30 per cent. This is powerful evidence of a causative role for *H. pylori*, although, as discussed later, problems with the side-effects of therapy have precluded the development of an acceptable regime which might form first-line treatment for duodenal ulcer disease.

RISK FACTORS FOR PEPTIC ULCER

Diet

Although dietary indiscretion has been widely accepted to be a cause of dyspepsia and peptic ulceration, there are few convincing studies clearly implicating dietary factors in causing or re-activating peptic ulceration. Conversely, it has been suggested that differences in diet may be responsible for some of the regional and international differences in the incidence and natural history of the disease; for example in the rice-eating belts of southern India duodenal ulcer is more common than in the wheat-eating areas in the north. In a Norwegian study duodenal ulcer recurrence rates were found to be higher in patients on a low-fibre diet, compared with people eating a normal or high-fibre diet.

Although not true causes of peptic ulceration, a number of drinks and foodstuffs are potent stimulants of acid secretion. Coffee, even when decaffeinated, is particularly effective, and beverages such as coke, fizzy lemonade, and beer are also potent stimulants, producing more than 50 per cent of the maximal acid secretory response seen with pentagastrin. Tea also stimulates gastric acid secretion, but none of these are thought to be specific risk factors for peptic ulcer disease. There is, however, evidence that the temperature at which tea and coffee drinkers prefer their beverages is high in peptic ulcer patients, implicating heat as a damaging factor.

Alcohol

Although concentrated alcohol applied directly to the gastric mucosa is a strong stimulant and can cause necrosis, there is no definite link between alcohol ingestion and peptic ulceration, despite the fact that most alcoholic beverages stimulate acid secretion. In some studies, duodenal ulcer patients were found to drink less alcohol than controls, presumably because alcohol may have an exacerbating effect on symptoms, and other studies suggest that moderate alcohol intake provides modest protection against duodenal ulceration. Alcoholics, paradoxically, are reported to be more prone to duodenal ulcer.

Drugs

Aspirin and other NSAIDs are now well known to cause not only acute gastric mucosal damage but also chronic ulceration, generally gastric, with its potential for perforation and haemorrhage. NSAID use has been firmly linked to the development of both gastric and duodenal ulcers. Endoscopic studies of arthritic patients taking these drugs generally reveal an excess of erosions and ulcers compared with control subjects, and retrospective studies of hospital in-patients show that NSAID ingestion is a relative risk factor for haemorrhage and perforation of both gastric and duodenal ulcers. It is also likely that NSAID-induced peptic ulceration is responsible for a number of sudden deaths related to haemorrhage or perforation in elderly patients.

Cigarette smoking

There is a clear association between smoking and duodenal ulcer disease. Epidemiological studies demonstrate that smokers are at increased risk for both duodenal and gastric ulcers, and data from several clinical trials show that smoking impairs the therapeutic response to a number of ulcer-healing drugs and also increases the risks of complications. There is a positive correlation in men and women between smoking trends and rates of death from duodenal ulcer disease. The mechanisms are uncertain, but the causative link is reasonably convincing.

Genetic factors

Three particular groups of data provide evidence for the existence of genetic factors in duodenal ulcer disease. These are the presence of familial aggregation, with 20–50 per cent of all duodenal ulcer patients having a positive family history, compared with 5–15 per cent in non-ulcer subjects, twin studies showing that concordance of peptic ulcer is more common in monozygotic than dizygotic twins, and the association between blood groups, HLA antigens, and secretor status. Individuals with blood group O have about a 30 per cent increase in risk of duodenal ulcer compared with those with other blood groups, and individuals who are not secretors of ABO blood group antigens have a 50 per cent increase in duodenal ulcer risk. There is some evidence linking specific HLA antigens, such as HLA-B_5 and HLA-B_{12}, with duodenal ulcer disease.

Additionally, there are a number of sub-types of familial duodenal ulcer disease, associated with specific syndromes including over-secretion of pepsinogen I, antral G-cell hyperfunction, childhood or early onset duodenal ulcer, and a syndrome of familial duodenal ulcer associated with rapid gastric emptying.

Finally, duodenal ulcer is linked to a number of rare genetic syndromes, including the multiple endocrine neoplasm syndrome (MEN) type I, systematic mastocytosis, type IV amyloidosis, and an extraordinary autosomal dominant condition called the tremor-nystagmus-ulcer syndrome.

Psychological factors

Psychodynamic factors in the genesis of duodenal ulcer disease have been investigated for many years, but their role remains controversial. A typical 'ulcer personality', characterized by an exaggerated dependency-independency conflict has been described, with exaggerated self-sufficiency acting as a defence mechanism against senses of shame and loss of confidence. Personality conflicts and duodenal ulcers were also linked in a study of 2000 army recruits and the degrees of dependency and conflict surrounding dependency were predictors of the development of duodenal ulcer in some of them.

Other compelling arguments have been articulated about the role of psychological stress in producing peptic ulcer disease. The blitz of London in 1941 was associated with an increase in perforated peptic ulcer rates, and other disaster research has suggested that stress may have adverse effects on the gastrointestinal tract. However, Scottish data from the Second World War have not supported this hypothesis. When considering the role of stress, illness onset has carefully to be distinguished from illness declaration; stressful life events may simply precipitate a medical consultation rather than the disease which is the subject of that consultation. However, there are plausible theories linking psychological factors to ulcer disease through changes in acid, pepsin, and mucus secretion and changes in gastric blood flow and motility. One model would suggest that psychodynamic predisposition and psychic conflict, coupled with unusual vulnerability to stressful life events may underly or exacerbate duodenal ulcer disease in some patients, with these factors acting through changes in aggressive and defensive gastric and duodenal mucosal mechanisms.

CLINICAL FEATURES

The classic description of duodenal ulcer disease included gnawing or burning epigastric pain occurring one to two hours after meals, but more quickly after a small, rather than a large, meal, frequently waking the patient at night, but rarely occurring before breakfast. The site of pain was said to be well demarcated, with the patient pointing a finger rather than placing the whole hand across the upper abdomen. Although some traditional texts state that the pain is located over a limited area and does not radiate unless penetration of the pancreas has occurred, more recent studies report that radiation of the pain into the back occurs in as many as 31 per cent of patients with duodenal ulcer. Rapid relief of the pain, at least in the early stages of ulceration, is obtained by eating, drinking milk, or taking alkaline preparations. Periodicity of pain is characteristic, with symptoms clustering for several days or weeks, followed by longer pain-free periods. For some reason, exacerbations are more common during the spring and autumn months.

Unfortunately, many of these 'typical' symptoms have poor specificity and sensitivity for distinguishing duodenal ulcer from other causes of epigastric discomfort. For example, only 31 per cent of patients presenting with epigastric pain who noted relief with food were found, on investigation, to have a duodenal ulcer as the underlying disorder. Night pain, however, is a much more significant feature, with higher specificity and sensitivity than most of the other typical symptoms. About one-half of all patients with duodenal ulcer do not, however, relate their pain to meals at all and occasionally pain occurs only with eating or within 30 minutes after eating. The classically-described increase in appetite is, in fact, seen in only about 20 per cent of patients with duodenal ulcer, with 45 per cent experiencing anorexia or even weight loss. Nausea and vomiting are common, occurring in between 25 and 60 per cent of patients with duodenal ulcer, and a variety of other dyspeptic symptoms occurring in between 40 and 70 per cent of cases. Heartburn, often with the characteristics of GORD, occurs in 20–60 per cent of patients with duodenal ulcer and a number of these subjects will also have symptoms typical of irritable bowel syndrome. The presence of this variable symptom-complex makes accurate and confident diagnosis on the basis of clinical symptoms alone hazardous.

The development of complications is likely to be associated with a change in symptoms. For example, when gastric outlet obstruction has developed patients may present with anorexia, weight loss, and vomiting after meals, often vomiting food ingested many hours earlier. Perforation and haemorrhage are less likely to be misdiagnosed.

A number of studies have shown that the simple model of an ulcer crater being bathed by acid is a poor explanation for the pain experienced by patients with duodenal ulcers. Ulcer healing does not guarantee disappearance of symptoms; although most patients who are shown at endoscopy to be ulcer-free are asymptomatic, as many as 39 per cent of ulcer-free patients report persistent symptoms. Ulcers may be present without producing any symptoms at all; the disappearance of symptoms by no means guarantees that the ulcer has healed and, conversely, the persistence of symptoms does not necessarily predict a persistent ulcer crater. Other factors are clearly involved in producing the pain of duodenal ulceration.

It is impossible, on the basis of the clinical history alone, to distinguish accurately between gastric and duodenal ulcer, which co-exist in about 7 per cent of patients. Characteristically, however, the pain of gastric ulcer is not relieved by food and may often be precipitated by eating. The typical periodicity seen in patients with duodenal ulcer is much less common in gastric ulcer disease.

Although uncommon, symptoms arising from postbulbar ulcers may be atypical, with patients reporting right upper quadrant or back pain only, little or no periodicity, and a disappointing response to antacid ingestion.

In children, in whom duodenal ulcers sometimes occur, atypical abdominal pain is often seen, with anorexia, vomiting, and unusual eating habits often reported. Recurrent vomiting can be a presentation of peptic ulcer in children. In the elderly, symptoms may, once again, be atypical; the pain may be less severe, the history shorter, and presentation with a complication of ulceration is not uncommon.

The main differential diagnoses in patients presenting with upper abdominal pain include a variety of abdominal problems, including gastro-oesophageal reflux, non-ulcer dyspepsia, oesophageal and gastric cancer, and Crohn's disease. In addition, up to a quarter of patients with biliary tract disease may present with epigastric pain without typical radiation through the right upper quadrant, and less common problems such as acute pancreatitis, intestinal ischaemia, and gastrointestinal infection should also be borne in mind.

INVESTIGATION

The decision to investigate patients with upper abdominal symptoms is not straightforward, and the evaluation of dyspeptic symptoms has been dealt with elsewhere in this book. The decisions to be made include the selection of patients for investigation, the timing of investigation in relation to the prescription of symptomatic or definitive therapy, and the choice of investigation. For practical purposes, investigation of patients with a provisional diagnosis of duodenal ulcer means the selection of either a double contrast barium meal examination or an upper gastrointestinal endoscopy.

Much has been written about the relative merits and disadvantages of these two investigations, but there is now little doubt that endoscopy is the best first-line investigation for the evaluation of upper abdominal symptoms. Sensitivity and specificity of this investigation for the detection of mucosal lesions are much better than those of radiology and, in relation to duodenal ulcer in particular, endoscopy has the great advantage of being able to distinguish duodenal scarring from active ulceration. Gastric ulcers always require biopsy to exclude malignancy, so that any gastric ulcer identified by radiology will require endoscopic biopsy as part of standard management.

Disadvantages of endoscopy include the possibility of transmission of infection between patients and hospital staff, with increasingly stringent requirements for disinfection of instruments between cases. However, most patients tolerate the procedure extremely well, often requiring minimal or no sedation, and there is no doubt that the elderly, for whom the contortions of a double contrast barium meal present something of a challenge, tolerate endoscopy well.

Barium X-ray appearances of duodenal ulcer are variable. An obvious ulcer crater may be seen or changes may be more subtle, including signs such as bulbar spasm, deformity of the pyloric cannel, blunting or loss of the fornices of the duodenal bulb, an irregular mucosal pattern, or a clover leaf deformity of the duodenal mucosa. False positive results can occur when barium is trapped between mucosal folds so that the configuration of a suspected ulcer crater must be seen to be constant on multiple X-rays taken from different positions. Ulcers less than 0.5 cm in diameter are difficult to detect reliably on barium studies, and it is also important to realize that the technique used, the skill and interest of the radiologist, and the ability of the patient to co-operate with the examination are all important determinants of the accuracy, sensitivity, and specificity of the barium meal in detecting peptic ulcers.

By contrast, the specificity of endoscopy is generally greater than 90 per cent and although enlarged folds and spasm may obscure ulcers at endoscopy, the use of anti-cholinergic agents to reduce duodenal spasm may increase the endoscopic yield. As already discussed, the ability directly to visualize the mucosae and to take biopsies means that for most patients endoscopy will be the preferred investigation, where available.

The procedure is, however, not without its complications, although these are rare. A large survey by the American Society for Gastrointestinal Endoscopy indicated a complication rate of 0.13 per cent; major complications included perforation (0.03 per cent), bleeding (0.03 per cent), cardiopulmonary complications (0.06 per cent), and infection (0.008 per cent). Overall, the procedure carries significant morbidity at a rate of 1 per 1000 examinations and a mortality rate of 1 per 10 000 examinations. Once again the complication rate is related to the conditions under which the examination is performed, in particular the amount of sedation required and used, and the pre-existing health of the population being examined.

General practitioners' choices between radiology and endoscopy are, however, limited. The procedures are not equally available in all parts of the country, with most general practitioners in, for example, the Oxford region having direct access to double contrast barium meals, compared with only 50–60 per cent in the Northern region. Open access to endoscopy also varies widely, with less than half all district hospitals providing such a service, of whom only about one quarter operate a 'genuine' open-access service, in which general practitioners can refer directly for endoscopy without intervention or assessment of their request by a hospital doctor.

Although follow-up endoscopy is not required for patients with duodenal ulcer disease, when symptom relief is used as the yardstick of therapeutic success, a second endoscopy is mandatory in patients with gastric ulcers. The reason for this is that even multiple biopsy techniques may miss areas of neoplasia, and failure to heal after appropriate therapy is an indication for a more determined search for malignancy in and around the ulcer crater.

Few other investigations are relevant in the evaluation of patients suspected of having duodenal ulcer disease. Haematological tests are unlikely to shed much light on the clinical picture, although the unexpected finding of anaemia might change the investigative focus; tests of liver function, are, similarly, unlikely to have specific value, unless unexpected abnormalities are turned up. Faecal occult blood testing is of no value in determining the presence of bleeding lesions of the upper gastrointestinal tract. Finally, controversy has surrounded the importance of testing for *Helicobacter pylori*. A number of tests for infection by this organism have been developed, including blood tests to seek the presence of antibodies, histological staining and examination of biopsy material, culture of biopsy material, and breath tests to meausre labelled CO_2 liberated by the organism's intense urease activity. Rapid endoscopy room tests have been developed, and have been shown to possess acceptable validity, but a recent consensus conference on *Helicobacter* and duodenal disease concluded that because the organism is almost invariably present in patients with duodenal ulcer, there is no need to test for it. The role of *H. pylori* and the importance of determining its presence and eradication may, of course, assume greater importance in patients with refractory or frequently relapsing duodenal ulcers, and may also become more relevant as resistance to conventionally used antibiotics develops.

MEDICAL TREATMENT

The pharmacological treatment of duodenal ulcer and gastric ulcer is very similar. Gastric ulcer requires follow-up investigation to assess healing, while duodenal ulcer can be managed without confirmatory investigations. The main difference in response of the two types of ulcer is one of time to healing. Gastric ulcers tend to heal more slowly than duodenal ulcers. An important principle of management is that the disease is generally not cured by a single course of treatment. The use of anti-*Helicobacter* therapy may change this principle, but at. the moment treatment should be considered in terms of acute healing and long-term management.

PHARMACOLOGICAL AGENTS AVAILABLE

Drugs which decrease or counteract acid secretion

Studies of gastric pH measured over 24 hours have shown that the healing rates of duodenal and gastric ulcer relate to three factors; the extent of inhibition of gastric secretion, duration of inhibition over 24 hours, and duration of treatment. For duodenal ulcer it has been shown that optimal healing rates are achieved when the gastric pH is maintained at about pH 3 for 18–20 hours. Increasing the pH beyond this level would not be expected to improve healing rates in duodenal ulcer over four weeks, but if treatment is continued for longer than a lower gastric pH provides satisfactory healing rates. For the healing of gastric ulcer the duration of treatment seems more important than the extent of inhibition of gastric secretion.

Antacids

Antacids neutralize gastric acid and raise the pH. This action may not be the only mechanism involved in their pharmacological activity. Aluminium hydroxide has been shown to increase the mucosal prostaglandin E2 level in rodents and it is possible that such a mechanism may be involved in the therapeutic effects in humans. The traditional view, however, is that antacids, by decreasing gastric acidity, redress the imbalance of aggressive versus protective factors and promote ulcer healing. Numerous clinical trials since the late 1970s have clearly shown that antacids are effective ulcer healing agents, particularly in duodenal ulcer. The initial trials used large doses of highly potent antacids and side-effects, notably diarrhoea with magnesium antacids, were frequent. It has subsequently become clear that lower doses of antacids are equally effective and four-week duodenal ulcer healing rates of between 70 and 85 per cent have been reported with moderate doses of antacids, (equivalent to 200 mmol neutralizing capacity). In studies comparing antacids with H_2-receptor antagonists significant differences have been unusual, suggesting that antacid use is as effective as other ulcer healing agents. There is no data on the long-term management of gastric ulceration with antacids, but two small studies have shown that low-dose antacids (Maalox TC two tablets twice a day) prolonged remission from duodenal ulcer as effectively as cimetidine (400 mg) at bedtime).

Adverse effects from antacids are well recognized, if infrequently considered.

Phosphate depletion and osteomalacia have been reported with aluminium-containing antacids. Diarrhoea associated with magnesium is a dose-related effect, and alkalosis is common but rapidly reversed in patients with normal renal function. A number of potential, but few important, drug interactions exist and patients using regular antacids should be advised to take other drugs two hours before or after the use of the antacid which may limit absorption of other agents.

Summary

Antacids are effective, they can be cheap, and have traditionally been the first-line therapy for patients with dyspepsia. Convenience and marketing pressure, rather than any deficiency in activity, has kept them from being the first-line treatment for peptic ulcer.

H_2-receptor antagonists

Four drugs have been licensed in the UK and a fifth is available in Europe. Cimetidine, ranitidine, nizatidine, and famotidine are all available in the UK. Roxatidine is not marketed in the UK. Experience is greatest with the first of these, cimetidine, marketed in 1976 (Smith Kline Beecham). As this was the first orally active H_2-receptor antagonist available it was extensively investigated. The original dose defined for the treatment of peptic ulcer aimed to decrease gastric acidity throughout a 24-hour period. The half-life of cimetidine is relatively short, (approximately two hours), and therefore the original dosage schedule was 200 mg three times a day and a further 400 mg was given at night before bed. This old-fashioned regimen has been superseded by the move to bedtime dosing. The pharmocodynamic effect of H_2-receptor antagonists is most obvious when gastric secretion is unstimulated by food, so that the drugs have been shown to have most marked effects when given at bedtime. However, it is clear that ulcer healing relates both to the extent of inhibition of gastric secretion and to its duration throughout a 24-hour period, as well as to the length of treatment, so that twice-daily H_2-antagonists are as effective as single night-time doses.

Important clinical differences between the different H_2-antagonists are few. For most patients it is reasonable to prescribe the cheaper alternative. Cimetidine binds to oxidative enzymes (cytochrome P450) in the liver, causing a mild inhibition of their activity. These enzymes, in turn, are involved in the metabolism of many other drugs and their inhibition can lead to significant drug interactions. Such interactions lead to an increase in the blood level of the drug concerned and to side-effects with those drugs which act within a narrow therapeutic window. The main problem drugs are phenytoin, warfarin, and theophylline, which in excess give rise to serious unpleasant unwanted effects. Clinically important drug interactions are rare, nevertheless, even with cimetidine.

Ranitidine also binds to cytochrome P450, but it does so much less avidly, and hence drug interactions are unlikely to occur. The same is true of the newer H_2-antagonists.

One drug interaction which works through a different mechanism has recently gained some notoriety. It has been shown that alcohol is metabolized initially by an enzyme present in the stomach, alcohol dehydrogenase. Any alcohol metabolized by this mechanism becomes unavailable for absorption. In both animal and human studies it has been shown that cimetidine inhibits the activity of gastric alcohol dehydrogenase and this interaction could lead to higher blood levels of alcohol in patients who drink. This could clearly be of importance in relation to the legal limits of alcohol for various activities, including driving. Data are inconclusive and no firm recommendations can presently be made. It does seem that cimetidine interacts with alcohol dehydrogenase and this may also be true of ranitidine and nizatidine, but the effect does not seem to be shared by famotidine. The importance of this interaction depends on the experimental circumstances. Men have more gastric alcohol dehydrogenase than do women, and hence, are more likely to be affected by any interaction. Food also stimulates alcohol dehydrogenase, so interactions may be most prevalent when alcohol ingestion occurs with or after food. Studies so far have not convincingly shown that there is an important increase in blood alcohol levels. Nevertheless, it seems reasonable to advise patients not to drink alcohol whilst using these drugs.

Gynaecomastia and impotence are unwanted effects which have, on occasions, been related to cimetidine use. The overall incidence of either of these events is small and only gynaecomastia has really been shown to be related to cimetidine. It is most likely to occur in patients on long-term, high-dose cimetidine. Gynaecomastia has also been reported in association with ranitidine and the mechanism is not clear. Cimetidine does interfere with androgen levels and has been shown to increase prolactin levels. Headache is another unwanted effect which is reported somewhat more commonly than one might expect, but a clear relationship to H_2-antagonist use has not evolved.

Duodenal ulcer healing rates of between 70 and 80 per cent can be expected after four weeks' treatment with any of the H_2-antagonists given in standard doses. After two months' therapy 90–95 per cent of ulcers would be expected to have healed. In gastric ulcer three months' treatment is required to achieve healing rates at this level. No clear advantage for any individual H_2-antagonist has been demonstrated. Maintenance treatment with H_2-antagonists has traditionally employed half the dose used for healing. This was always an arbitrary decision, and it is clear that higher doses may be more effective at maintaining remission. Nevertheless, 400 mg of cimetidine and 150 mg of ranitidine have been shown to reduce the spontaneous relapse rate of duodenal ulcer from an expectation of 80 per cent per year to around 20 per cent per year. Two large studies have suggested that the more potent inhibitor of acid secretion, ranitidine, is associated with lower relapse rates than cimetidine. The need for maintenance treatment is debated, and indeed, it is unknown what proportion of ulcer patients at any one time are taking long-term therapy. There is a little evidence to suggest that long-term treatment does protect patients from complications of duodenal ulcer, but the data are not strong. Taking treatment *ad lib* when symptoms recur may be the way many patients deal with their disease, but firm evidence to support such therapy is lacking.

H_2-receptor antagonists remain first-line therapy for duodenal and gastric ulcer but cannot be considered curative (see *Helicobacter pylori*, p. 106). There is no evidence to suggest that this form of anti-secretory therapy eradicates *Helicobacter pylori*, and therefore a relapse following an acute course of treatment is expected. It has even been suggested that relapse rates following H_2-antagonists may be higher than normal through mild rebound acid hypersecretion which has been demonstrated in some studies. There is also a possibility that treatment with H_2-antagonists results in 'up-regulation' of H_2-receptors making them more sensitive to stimulants (and less sensitive to antagonists). A clinical connection between 'up-regulation' and relapse has been hypothesized but remains unproven. Another possible result of these factors is the development of tolerance, whereby the anti-secretory effect becomes less marked over time. This pharmacological effect is well recognized for many drugs which act at receptor sites, such as opiates, and there is some evidence to suggest that it occurs in human volunteers receiving H_2-receptor antagonists. An alternative explanation is that gastrin levels rise during therapy, resulting in greater background stimulation of acid secretion with time. No clinical significance has been demonstrated, irrespective of the mechanism, though it is possible that the increasing acidity which has been shown during treatment with H_2-antagonists could explain the relatively poor symptomatic response to these drugs in reflux oesophagitis.

Summary

H_2-antagonists are effective, safe, and are generally first-line treatments for peptic ulcer. No single H_2-antagonist clearly outshines the others. The drugs are useful for acute healing and long-term maintenance therapy.

Muscarinic antagonists

Traditional anticholinergic agents have not found favour in the management of peptic ulcer despite their moderate ability to decrease acid secretion. The older anti-cholinergic agents were non-specific in their action and produced the well-recognized side-effects of blurred vision, dry mouth, and urinary retention. Pirenzepine was the first more specific muscarinic antagonist; it aims to decrease gastric acid secretion without producing major side-effects. Studies have clearly shown that pirenzepine is an effective anti-secretory drug, though it has more effect on the volume of secretions than on their pH. Standard anti-cholinergic side-effects are unusual when the dose of 50 mg twice daily is used, but increase in frequency with increasing dosage. The drug has been much less extensively investigated than the H_2-antagonists, but trial data suggest that it is as effective in the healing of both duodenal and gastric ulcer in a dose of 50 mg twice daily. There is a small amount of evidence to suggest that long-term treatment with 50 mg pirenzepine at night is effective over a year in reducing relapse rates in duodenal ulcer.

Summary

Pirenzepine is an effective anti-ulcer agent with no particular virtues compared with other available drugs. The potential for side-effects has probably relegated it to second- or third-line therapy.

Hydrogen potassium ATPase inhibitors

Omeprazole was the first proton pump inhibitor to be marketed worldwide. Other drugs are in development and lansoprazole is likely to be the second agent to become available. These drugs differ from all other anti-secretory agents in that they inhibit the activity of the hydrogen potassium ATPase pump, which exchanges potassium ions from the lumen for hydrogen ions and is the final mechanism whereby hydrogen ions are secreted from parietal cells. It is clear, therefore, that inhibition of this enzyme results in a decreased acid secretory capacity irrespective of the mode of stimulation.

The studies with omeprazole have shown that it is the most potent orally active gastric anti-secretory agent available; lansoprazole appears to have equal potency. Both of these drugs require activation and are acid sensitive. To protect them from gastric acid they are presented as enteric-coated granules. These release their contents in the small intestine and after absorption the drug is concentrated in acid spaces. This means that it becomes concentrated in the parietal cells, where it is then activated and can block the action of the proton pump. A feature of these drugs is that their activity increases over the first few days and after stopping the agent acidity returns to normal after a few days. Doses of 20–40 mg of either agent produce a rise in gastric pH which is an order of magnitude greater than that achieved with the H_2-antagonists. Median 24-hour pH on proton pump inhibitors is around five, compared with 1.7 to 2.5 with the H_2-antagonists.

The development of these agents has been hampered by a serious toxicological problem in rodents. Omeprazole given life-long to rats resulted in hypertrophy of endocrine cells in the stomach. These particular cells, (enterochromaffin like, ECL, cells), are present in large numbers in the rat but in small numbers in man. They are more frequently found in female rats than male rats. Their growth appears to be controlled in part by gastrin and in rodents, at least, they contain granules of histamine and may be involved in the control of acid secretion at the parietal cell.

A proportion of the rats treated life-long developed carcinoid tumours of these cells which did not metastasize. There is a large body of data to suggest that the ECL cell hyperplasia and ECL cell carcinoids in rats are a result of hypergastrinaemia secondary to potent anti-secretory therapy. In support of this is evidence that if the gastrin-secreting cells are removed, ECL carcinoids do not occur in rats treated with omeprazole. Further support comes from studies using high-dose H_2-antagonists which have shown that ECL hyperplasia is also a feature of such treatment. Once the explanation for these changes became clearer, development of the drugs was allowed to proceed.

It is not known whether humans might respond similarly to the rat. ECL carcinoids have been reported in humans associated with pernicious anaemia, (with very high levels of gastrin), and with Zollinger–Ellison syndrome, (a gastrin-secreting tumour). When ECL cell carcinoids have been found in patients with pernicious anaemia they have tended to behave in a relatively benign fashion and some have been shown to regress spontaneously. It is impossible at this stage to categorically declare that such a problem would not arise from continuous treatment with proton pump inhibitors in humans. It seems likely that hypergastrinaemia of an order of magnitude greater than that which occurs usually in patients taking proton pump inhibitors would need to be present for many years before such changes could be anticipated.

This fact needs to be considered when long-term treatment with proton pump inhibitors is considered in quite young people who are likely to require treatment for 10–20 years. Nevertheless, certain groups of people do require and indeed benefit greatly from long-term proton pump inhibition.

The relationship of ulcer healing to anti-secretory treatment is reasonably well understood. Raising intragastric pH to levels of 3 or greater provides optimum treatment if this level of pH is maintained for 18–20 hours. It is not surprising, therefore, that ulcer healing trials comparing omeprazole and lansoprazole with H_2-antagonists have shown an advantage to the proton pump inhibitors. Following two weeks' treatment approximately 70 per cent of duodenal ulcers are healed with the proton pump inhibitors and at four weeks ulcer healing rates approximate to 90 per cent. These healing rates are similar to those achieved with H_2-antagonists given for twice as long. The advantage in gastric ulcer is not as great as that in duodenal ulcer. The proton pump inhibitors have been shown to be particularly effective in relieving symptoms and healing the lesions of reflux oesophagitis. The standard dose of omeprazole is 20–40 mg daily and for lansoprazole is 30 mg daily. There is insufficient data on long-term maintenance treatment with either of these agents to recommend their use in long-term treatment of peptic ulcer. The expectation is that they would be highly effective.

Summary

The proton pump inhibitors are the most potent anti-secretory agents presently available. Powerful suppression of acid secretion is associated with rapid ulcer healing and it would not be unreasonable if these agents became first-line anti-secretory therapy. Experience with them is limited compared with the H_2-antagonists.

Drugs which do not affect gastric secretion

Three agents have been available for treatment of peptic ulcer whose mechanisms of action are poorly understood. They do not affect gastric acid secretion and they are therefore believed to improve the defensive capacity of the mucosa to withstand injury. Mechanisms suggested include stimulation of mucus and bicarbonate secretion, protein binding providing a physical barrier and anti-*Helicobacter* activity. The latter is of greatest interest in view of the suggestion that duodenal ulceration at least might be cured by eradication of *Helicobacter*.

Sucralfate

This drug is a sulphated aluminium salt of sucrose. It appears to increase endogenous prostaglandin synthesis and production of mucus. It binds to the protein base of an ulcer crater and through these mechanisms may protect the damaged mucosa from further injury. In theory, this binding only takes place in the presence of acid, but in practice many patients probably use sucralfate together with antacids.

Controlled studies have demonstrated that 1 g four times daily is as effective as the H_2-receptor antagonists in the treatment of both duodenal and gastric ulcer. Less frequent dosing may be effective but few trials have been performed. Side-effects are minimal and are limited to the occasional episode of constipation.

Summary

Sucralfate is an effective anti-ulcer agent but requires multiple dosing. The tablets are large.

Carbenoxolone sodium

This was one of the earliest ulcer treatments available. Its mode of action is not understood, but is has aldosterone-like activity and stimulates gastric mucus production. Placebo-controlled trials demonstrated that it was effective, but few comparative studies with the H_2-antagonists have been performed. Side-effects have been a problem and its use has generally been superseded by the newer drugs. Serious side-effects include sodium retention, leading to hypertension, oedema, and hypokalaemia. The therapeutic activity of carbenoxolone is negated by the aldosterone antagonist spironolactone, which suggests that its activity is somehow related to aldosterone-like effects.

Summary

Carbenoxolone can not be recommended for routine use in view of the significant side-effects and the free availability of other safer agents.

Bismuth compounds

The most common bismuth agent used is tripotassium dicitratobismuthate (De-Nol, colloidal bismuth). It forms an insoluble mixture with proteins at the base of ulcers and results in a protective barrier. This may be the underlying mechanism for its ulcer healing actions. One other property of bismuth may be more important and relates to anti-*Helicobacter pylori* activity. *In-vitro* bismuth salts are bactericidal to *Helicobacter*, though *in-vivo* eradication of *Helicobacter* is unusual following bismuth alone.

Single therapy

Trials have shown conclusively that colloidal bismith in liquid and tablet form produces ulcer-healing rates equivalent to those achieved with the H_2-antagonists. The doses of the tablet formulation used are one tablet four times a day or two tablets twice daily (De-Nol tabs). There is also some evidence to suggest that ulcers which fail to respond to cimetidine heal on further courses of De-Nol. There is little data on long-term therapy with De-Nol, but the small studies which have been done suggest that it is effective.

Duodenal ulcer relapse rates following healing with De-Nol are lower than those after H_2-antagonist therapy. There are two potential mechanisms to explain this effect. First, bismuth seems to remain in the body for many weeks after a single course of treatment. Urine bismuth levels rise and remain high long after treatment has been stopped. It has been suggested that this represents a depot of bismuth somewhere (possibly in the gastrointestinal mucosa) which allows it to continue to offer a therapeutic effect even when treatment has been stopped. The second and more likely explanation relates to its anti-*Helicobacter* effect. It is recognized that *Helicobacter pylori* is suppressed following a course of bismuth, but in most patients the organism returns four weeks or so after the treatment has been stopped. Around 20 per cent of patients may have true eradication following De-Nol alone. It is possible, therefore, that suppression of *Helicobacter* also suppresses relapse of duodenal ulcer. There is good evidence that true eradication of *Helicobacter* renders ulcer relapse most unlikely (p. 107).

Eradication of *Helicobacter pylori*

Eradication has come to be defined as the absence of *Helicobacter pylori* one month after stopping a course of ulcer-healing treatment. As discussed above, certain treatments may suppress *Helicobacter pylori* but individual agents rarely eradicate the organism. Lansoprazole, omeprazole, and De-Nol have all been shown to suppress the organism, but true eradication requires the use of more than one drug. Various regimens have evolved using two, three or four agents for varying periods. The numbers of patients with successful eradication around the world remain quite small, but increasing evidence suggests that following eradication duodenal ulcers do not relapse unless the patient acquires a further infection with

Table 7.1 *One-week treatment regimen for eradication of Helicobacter pylori. (After Logan, R. P. H. et al. (1991). Lancet,* **2**, *1249–52.)*

DeNoltabs—1 four times daily for one week.
Amoxycillin—500 mg four times daily for one week.
Metronidazole—400 mg five times daily for the last three days of the week.
Medication taken concurrently and patients warned not to take alcohol.

Helicobacter. It is believed that the spontaneous infection rate approximates to 1 per cent per year, and therefore relapse rates following true eradication should be of this order.

The regimens used have been shown to produce eradication rates of between 60 and 80 per cent. The most common drug combinations include a bismuth compound, a broad-spectrum antibiotic (amoxycillin or tetracycline), metronidazole or tinidazole, and in some an anti-secretory agent is included. The use of broad-spectrum antibiotics has led to occasional reports of pseudo-membranous colitis, and drug reactions with antibiotics are not uncommon. Thus the present regimens cannot be recommended for routine ulcer therapy, but patients with particularly frequent and troublesome recurrences, as well as those with repeated symptomless complications, should probably be offered at least one attempt to eradicate the organism. Failure to produce eradication is said to be due to resistance of the organism to metronidazole, though a proportion of failures occur even with regimens that do not include this drug. A one-week treatment regimen for eradication of *Helicobacter pylori* has been published (Table 7.1). This regimen is shown as an example, but simpler and possibly better tolerated drug regimens are under investigation and firm recommendations cannot be made at this stage.

Summary

Denol is an effective ulcer therapy and relapse rates are lower following healing. Alone it does not eradicate *Helicobacter pylori* in many, but it forms part of many regimens including antibiotics for this purpose.

Drugs which combine inhibition of gastric secretion with mucosal protection

Prostaglandins

Misoprostol is a synthetic analogue of prostaglandin E1 and is the first prostaglandin to be marketed for ulcer therapy. In common with other prostaglandins of the E series it decreases gastric secretion. In addition, these prostaglandins have multiple other effects which participate in mucosal protection. The ability of these drugs to protect the mucosa at doses which do not inhibit acid secretion led to the term cytoprotection. Amongst these mechanisms are increasing mucus and bicarbonate secretion and increasing mucosal blood flow. The relationship between protection of acute injury and ulcer healing is tenous and cytoprotection may be unimportant in ulcer therapy.

The stimulation of gastrointestinal motility which prostaglandins tend to produce has limited their development. Diarrhoea is a recognized side-effect of misoprostol, but this problem does not often lead to withdrawal of therapy. It is usually self-limiting despite continuing treatment. Misoprostol may also induce abortion and is therefore contra-indicated in women of childbearing potential and in pregnancy. There are occasional reports of post-menopausal bleeding in patients receiving misoprostol.

Misoprostol, 200 μg four times daily or 400 μg twice daily, has been shown to be an effective gastric and duodenal ulcer-healing agent. Healing rates equate to those achieved with other anti-ulcer drugs and there is no suggestion that misoprostol is more effective than other agents. As simple ulcer therapy it can be considered an effective second- or third-line agent in view of the more frequent side-effects associated with it. There is insufficient data on maintenance therapy with misoprostol.

A particular role for misoprostol has been suggested in the prevention and therapy of ulcers associated with non-steroidal anti-inflammatory drugs. Two large studies in patients on long terms NSAIDs have shown that concomitant use of misoprostol can prevent the development of acute gastric and duodenal ulceration. There are various schools of thought about which patients (if any) should receive such 'prophylaxis'. One problem with NSAIDs is the development of abdominal symptoms and it has not been shown that misoprostol can prevent such symptoms. The most serious events associated with non-steroidal use are the complications (perforation and bleeding) from duodenal and gastric ulcer. There is, as yet, no evidence to suggest that misoprostol can prevent these serious adverse events. Further studies are underway and recommendations about when or if to use misoprostol at all will follow their results.

Summary

Misoprostol combines mucosal protection with suppression of gastric acid. It is an effective ulcer-healing agent, but it's side-effects are more frequent than with H_2-receptor antagonists. A definite role in non-steroidal associated ulceration requires further evidence.

THE PHILOSOPHY OF ULCER TREATMENT

Numerous agents are equally effective at healing ulcers in the short term. Most ulcer patients suffer repeated relapses and it is their long-term management which is most difficult and costly. Until simple and safe *Helicobacter* eradication regimens become available (and assuming eradication does produce cure) strategies have to be developed for each individual. The alternatives are repeated single courses of treatment for each relapse, long-term continuous treatment (maintenance), *ad-lib* therapy, or surgery. Firm scientific data is only available for the first two alternatives. *Ad-lib* therapy has been inadequately studied but many believe it to be the way patients manage their own ulcers. Surgery has a place in some patients, usually for individual reasons. Surgery also has a major role to play in treating complications of peptic ulceration. Patients should be offered a choice of all these strategies to aid decision-making and compliance. In economic terms *ad-lib* therapy is the cheapest alternative, but the costs of maintenance therapy and surgery are probably equivalent in the long run. Cure is clearly the most desirable result from any therapy and here anti-*Helicobacter* treatment may play an important role in the future.

Summary

Firm recommendations about long-term therapy must take account of patient preference. Maintenance therapy or surgery will prevent recurrence in most but may be unacceptable to many. 'Cure' by eradication of *Helicobacter* is a distinct future possibility.

FURTHER READING

Kurata, J. H. and Haile, B. M. (1984). Epidemiology of peptic ulcer disease. *Clinical Gastroenterology*, **13**, 289–307.

Kurata, J. H., Nogawa, A. N., Abbey, D. E. and Petersen, F. (1992). A prospective study of risk for peptic ulcer disease in Seventh-Day Adventists. *Gastroenterology*, **102**, 902–9.

Langman, M. J. S. (1989). Epidemiologic evidence on the association between peptic ulceration and anti-inflammatory drug use. *Gastroenterology*, **96**, 640–6.

Moss, S. and Calam, J. (1992). *Helicobacter pylori* and peptic ulcers: the present position. *Gut*, **33**, 289–92.

Penston, J. G. and Wormsley, K. G. (1992). Maintenance treatment with H_2-receptor antagonists for peptic ulcer disease. *Alimentary Pharmacology and Therapeutics*, **6**, 3–30.

Tibblin, G. (1985). Introduction to the epidemiology of dyspepsia. *Scandinavican Journal of Gastroenterology*, **20**, (Suppl. 109) 29–33.

Walker, P., Luther, J., Samloff, I. M. and Feldman, M. (1988). Life events stress and psychosocial factors in men with peptic ulcer disease: relationships with serum pepsinogen concentrations and behavioural risk factors. *Gastroenterology*, **94**, 323–30.

8 Functional bowel disorders

Richard Stevens and Roger Jones

Patients with gastroenterological symptoms for which no pathophysio-logical cause can be found are as least as common in clinical practice as those with symptoms for which a cause is established. The spectrum of 'functional disorders' include non-ulcer dyspepsia if the symptoms are predominantly in the upper gastrointestinal tract and irritable bowel syndrome if the symptoms are lower gastrointestinal. This chapter will focus largely on irritable bowel syndrome, non-ulcer dyspepsia being dealt with in Chapter 3.

Patients with symptoms of irritable bowel syndrome are seen frequently in general practice and in gastroenterological clinics, where 50 per cent of patients are eventually found to have a functional diagnosis. Add to this number those patients seen as surgical and gynaecological outpatients and it is clear that the functional bowel disorders have profound clinical and resource implications.

In the past it has been stated that irritable bowel syndrome is a diagnosis of exclusion, but more recently it has become clear that it is possible to make a positive diagnosis based on the patient's history. It is interesting to speculate on the basis of many general practitioners' reluctance to make a clinical diagnosis on a classic history in the case of irritable bowel syndrome. The same general practitioners are usually happy to diagnose and treat conditions such as asthma, migraine, and angina pectoris on the basis of the history alone.

There are considerable benefits for patients in irritable bowel syndrome being a positive diagnosis. In many cases they can be spared unpleasant, invasive, and expensive investigations. There is also a group of patients who are wrongly labelled as suffering from irritable bowel syndrome purely because investigations of their lower gastrointestinal tract are normal.

FUNCTIONAL BOWEL SYMPTOMS IN THE COMMUNITY

The various combinations of chronic or recurrent gastrointestinal symptoms to which diagnoses of 'functional disorder' are assigned in the hospital clinic are also extremely common in the general population, where the majority of patients do not consult doctors about them. A number of studies have described the prevalence and pattern of these disorders in the general population and have also estimated, using the Manning criteria, which are described later, the prevalence of irritable bowel syndrome in the community. Many of the early population-based studies were flawed by inadequate randomization and the choice of atypical populations, but two recent studies have provided information from large, randomized samples from the general population.

In the first of these, from Southampton, a validated postal questionnaire was sent to more than 2000 patients, in whom a variety of symptoms were reported in the previous 12 months, including diarrhoea (22 per cent), constipation (21 per cent), the passage of mucus per rectum (12 per cent), rectal bleeding (15 per cent), and recurrent abdominal pain (25 per cent). The one-year prevalence of irritable bowel syndrome amongst these patients was 21.6 per cent.

In a study from the Mayo Clinic, USA, a questionnaire was also used to survey bowel symptoms in more than 1000 residents of Olmsted County. The prevalence of abdominal pain on more than six occasions in the previous year was identical to the British survey (25 per cent), and figures for other symptoms were remarkably similar—constipation 17 per cent, diarrhoea 18 per cent, the passage of mucus 16 per cent, and blood on the toilet paper 13 per cent. In this study the one-year prevalence of irritable bowel syndrome as defined by the Manning criteria was 17 per cent.

In both of these studies, the majority of subjects had not sought medical advice about their problems, and the likelihood that they would consult was not accounted for by differences in symptom frequency or severity.

DEFINING IRRITABLE BOWEL SYNDROME

Reaching a universal definition of irritable bowel syndrome has proved to be an elusive goal. Often comparisons cannot be made between different studies as different definitions of the condition are used. The standard definition as 'abdominal pain and altered bowel habit not due to organic disease' has been replaced by an International Working Party's definition 'variable but characteristic combination of symptoms attributable to disordered function of the intestine with no demonstrable structural or biochemical cause'. This, of course, begs the question as to what exactly are the *characteristic* combinations of symptoms.

The most commonly agreed symptom-set used in the definition and diagnosis of irritable bowel syndrome are those described by Manning in 1978. By using a questionnaire to record symptoms in unselected patients attending hospital out-patient departments and looking for features which discriminated those patients whose final diagnosis was of irritable bowel syndrome from those who finally had an organic disease diagnosis, four predictors of a functional diagnosis were distinguished, as follows:

(1) visible abdominal distension;
(2) relief of pain with bowel movement;
(3) more frequent bowel movements with the onset of pain;
(4) loose stools at onset of pain.

The greater the number of these four symptoms that were present the greater the likelihood of the diagnosis of irritable bowel syndrome. Two further symptoms were also found to discriminate the two groups, although with less accuracy:

(5) passage of mucus per rectum;
(6) feeling of incomplete evacuation.

Long-term follow-up studies have confirmed the reliability and discriminatory value of the Manning criteria. These tend to confirm that patients can be safely diagnosed on clinical grounds, and that organic disease can be discriminated from functional disease on the basis of those cardinal symptoms. Given the high prevalence of irritable bowel syndrome symptoms in the community and the concurrent relatively high rates of colo-rectal neoplasm, especially in the older age group, some patients clearly still warrant investigation. However, a great many others, predominately in the younger age group, can be safely diagnosed and treated, on the basis of the Manning criteria. Not only does posing the correct question aid the doctor in making a diagnosis, but if the answers are largely positive his or her credibility with the patient is increased.

Two further studies support the contention that irritable bowel syndrome can be distinguished from organic bowel disease on the basis of symptoms alone. The Mayo clinic group have developed a 46-item questionnaire that discriminates functional from organic bowel disease with a sensitivity of 85 per cent and a specificity of 60 per cent. Although the use of such questionnaires is uncommon in clinical practice, the finding does serve to emphasize the fact that there is a set of symptoms which, if present, can be used to arrive at a positive diagnosis of irritable bowel syndrome. Likewise, logistic regression has been used in the analysis of over 700 patients in Glasgow with a variety of gastroenterological conditions to produce a list of 13 symptoms commonly found in those patients diagnosed as having irritable bowel syndrome. These symptoms are:

(1) history of abdominal pain in childhood;
(2) previous emergency treatment sought for severe pain;
(3) episodic pain;

 (4) pain relieved by bowel motion;
 (5) abnormal bowel function;
 (6) pain induced by purgation;
 (7) diarrhoea induced by pain;
 (8) alternating diarrhoea and constipation;
 (9) episodic diarrhoea and constipation;
(10) pebble-like stools and abdominal pain;
(11) mucus in stool.

Clearly there is overlap with the better established Manning criteria which, if only by virtue of their brevity, are largely sufficient for everyday practice.

One caveat about all the work done on symptom discrimination in irritable bowel syndrome is that the studies almost always use populations of hospital out-patients. There is evidence to suggest that patients who are referred tend to have worse symptoms and greater anxiety levels than patients in general practice. Nevertheless, the emerging view that irritable bowel syndrome can be a safe clinical diagnosis is to the benefit of both clinicians and patients.

SYMPTOMS ASSOCIATED WITH IRRITABLE BOWEL SYNDROME

A number of non-colonic symptoms are known to be associated with irritable bowel syndrome. The change in name from 'spastic colon' to irritable bowel syndrome acknowledges the pan-gut nature of the condition, and perhaps a further change in title is indicated given the increasing recognition of the involvement of other symptoms. These associated symptoms have given rise to speculation as to the aetiology of the condition and in particular to the notion that irritable bowel syndrome is part of a generalized disorder of smooth muscle. This remains speculative at present, and other theories promote the view that the symptoms are due to increased perception of somatic sensations in affected individuals, or that sufferers are a group of 'chronic complainers' in whom multi-system symptoms can be expected.

Non-ulcer dyspepsia, especially with features of nausea and vomiting, dysphagia, early satiety, and excessive flatus is found more commonly in patients diagnosed as having irritable bowel syndrome. If these symptoms co-exist with the more classic features of irritable bowel syndrome it is hardly surprising that there is often diagnostic uncertainty. Similarly, the reported higher incidence of rectal bleeding can be another alarming and confusing factor. One explanation for this last fact may be the known association between the stool inspection and reporting of rectal bleeding.

Stool inspection rates could perhaps be expected to be higher in patients with bowel disturbances. Abnormalities of gall-bladder contraction and sensitivity to cholecystokinins have also been reported in certain classes of patients with irritable bowel syndrome.

The association of urinary symptoms—frequency, urgency, hesitancy, and incomplete emptying of the bladder—with irritable bowel syndrome have given rise to the notion of an irritable bladder syndrome with a similar pathogenesis. These urinary symptoms can lead to the incorrect diagnosis of recurrent urinary tract infection and unnecessary investigations.

Women sufferers with irritable bowel syndrome report an increased incidence of dyspareunia. In one hospital-based study, the reported incidence of dyspareunia was greater than 70 per cent. Typically, the pain occurred after intercourse. Gynaecologists are increasingly making the diagnosis of irritable bowel syndrome and earlier recognition of associated symptoms by general practitioners could lead, at least, to more appropriate referral. Interestingly, there is no reported increased incidence of dysmenorrhoea or premenstrual tension in patients with irritable bowel syndrome. This would seem to argue against the theory that patients with irritable bowel syndrome are merely a group of 'chronic complainers'.

The smooth muscle of the lungs is also more reactive in patients with irritable bowel syndrome. In a small study it has been shown that there is a greater bronchial reactivity in the face of a methacholine challenge in patients with irritable bowel syndrome compared with normal controls.

Migraine has also been found to occur with greater frequency in patients with irritable bowel syndrome. Again, this is used as further evidence for the generalized disorder of smooth muscle theory; in this case the smooth muscle of the cranial vessels is thought of as being hyper-active.

Various non-specific symptoms have also been described in association with irritable bowel syndrome. These are lack of energy, back pain, an unpleasant taste in the mouth, and poor sleep. The vagueness of these complaints makes their significance hard to interpret, and conceivably could be related to disordered bowel motility—a constant feature in irritable bowel syndrome.

PATIENT BEHAVIOUR: CONSULTATION FOR IRRITABLE BOWEL SYNDROME

Symptoms of irritable bowel syndrome in the community are common, although accurate prevalence studies have proved notoriously difficult. The major difficulties are subject selection of people who are not attending a health professional, and an agreed definition of what constitutes irritable bowel syndrome. Studies both from the UK and the USA give prevalence figures ranging from 13.6 to 26 per cent.

A potential methodological bias is that these studies use questionnaires or structured interviews which depend on accurate recall and admission of symptoms. These symptoms will be more memorable, and therefore more easily recalled, by patients who have high levels of concern about them. There is some evidence that when subjects are asked to record their symptoms prospectively that apparently similar symptoms occur with similar frequencies in those who had initially denied suffering from such symptoms. These symptom-deniers or symptom-tolerators presumably do not remember them or think them worthy of recall subsequently.

It can be speculated that the weight an individual attaches to their symptoms also affects the likelihood of them contacting a doctor. Only a minority of symptomatic patients seek medical advice (33 per cent in a large study in the south of England). Symptom severity did not seem to be associated with consultation behaviour, but factors such as an individual's general practitioner and the presence of other symptoms, notably rectal bleeding, did affect the likelihood of consulting. Studies of dyspepsia and consultation behaviour have demonstrated that it is not always symptom severity or frequency, but specific health concerns about their symptoms, that brings patients to the doctor, and a similar situation exists with irritable bowel syndrome.

In an interview study of patients identified in a community survey as having irritable bowel syndrome, those who consulted a general practitioner were much more concerned about the potential 'seriousness' of their symptoms than those who did not: the non-consulting group were often positively dismissive about their symptoms and regarded them as variations of normal. The consulting group also contained an excess of patients with abnormal scores for anxiety and depression on the Hospital Anxiety and Depression scale. The widely held view of increased neuroticism in irritable bowel syndrome sufferers may also be a reflection of consultation behaviour. The subset of sufferers with anxiety produced by their bowel symptoms that results in their consulting may not be representative of all sufferers in the community. The place of psychological factors in irritable bowel syndrome has been a topic of controversy for some years, but the stereotype of a disorder of neurotic middle-aged women has finally been abandoned. It is clear from work in the UK and the USA that psychological factors are associated not with irritable bowel syndrome in itself, but with the decision to seek medical advice. A thorough prospective study of 97 patients attending a gastroenterology clinic in North Carolina evaluated a wide range of psychosocial variables, including anxiety, depression, stress, social support, somatization, and abnormal illness behaviour. These factors were not associated with a final diagnosis of functional, as opposed to organic, bowel disease, but were determinants of health care seeking for patients, irrespective of their final diagnosis.

If psychosocial factors are important determinants of the decision to consult, does the severity of symptoms also predict those patients likely to seek medical advice? There is evidence that consulting patients do indeed have more pain and more troublesome bowel symptoms than non-consulting subjects, and the interview study from Southampton mentioned earlier also showed significantly more painful abdominal distension in the consulting group. In a further study of hospital out-patients from Manchester, the characteristics of first time and chronic clinic attenders with irritable bowel syndrome were compared. The chronic attenders perceived their colonic and non-colonic symptoms as more severe than the first time attenders, were more likely to complain of constant, unremitting symptoms and to find that their symptoms had more disruptive social consequences. Psychiatric morbidity was similar and substantial (49 per cent and 45 per cent) in both groups, suggesting once again that observations made in the hospital setting are often representative of a selected patient population.

Are patients who consult with abdominal symptoms and are given a diagnosis of irritable bowel syndrome more 'sensitive' to changes in visceral sensations than normal? This has been a subject of considerable research interest which has generated a large volume of often conflicting data, which are often difficult to compare because of the different experimental methods used. There is, however, reasonable evidence of disturbed ano-rectal function and sensation in irritable bowel syndrome, which has different patterns in diarrhoea-predominant and constipation-predominant patients. The threshold for perception of intestinal contraction is lower, at least in some patients with irritable bowel syndrome, and visceral pain sensitivity may also be increased: there is no consensus about whether the mechanisms involved are peripheral or central. The abdominal distension of irritable bowel syndrome remains a mystery and the argument that it is related to changes in motility or tone of gastrointestinal smooth muscle is not entirely convincing.

A further distorting factor in producing the relatively large number of patients seen in gastroenterology out-patients clinics—the most widely studied sample of patients with irritable bowel syndrome—is the general practitioner's decision to refer. Only about 1 in 7 patients are referred for specialist opinion and little is known about the factors influencing the decision to refer.

TREATMENT OF IRRITABLE BOWEL SYNDROME

To establish an objective of treatment it is important to determine whether an individual patient has consulted primarily on account of their symptoms and the impact they are having on their life, or because of the anxiety-inducing interpretation they have attached to them. In the latter case the patient may not have conscious awareness that it is fear of serious or unknown disease that is the basis of their distress. Many patients will, of course, be concerned on both counts.

The studies that demonstrate that consulting patients with irritable bowel syndrome differ only in their health-seeking behaviour and not in the severity of their symptoms would indicate that explanation and reassurance may be the most appropriate treatment for many people. The majority of irritable bowel syndrome sufferers are content to accept their symptoms as a feature of their life, and perhaps the group of consulters may also do so if their concerns as to the implications of their symptoms were to be addressed. It is clearly of great importance that the patient's symptoms are taken seriously by the general practitioner, who is prepared to take a full and sympathetic history and to undertake a reasonably thorough physical examination. This reassures the patient that nothing has been overlooked. Patients clearly should be encouraged to discuss and understand their fears about the significance of their symptoms, so that they can be dealt with as soon as the general practitioner feels sufficiently confident to do so.

Explanation of the way that symptoms are produced may also be important and helpful in management. Discomfort and bloating confined to the upper abdomen may be due to distension of the transverse colon, and this could be pointed out to patients. Descriptions of the colicky pain that can arise from distension or spasm in the gut, or discussion of disordered bowel activity leading to altered bowel habit may also help the patient to understand the complexities of the symptoms. Some gastro-enterologists use rigid sigmoidoscopy and air insufflation to reproduce the pain experienced by patients, in an attempt to demonstrate the mechanical, as opposed to sinister, nature of the pain.

Providing acceptable reassurance on a diagnosis made almost exclusively on the basis of a typical history can, however, be difficult for some doctors. Uneasiness in the doctor about the diagnosis, particularly concern about missing serious disease, may prevent fulsome and credible reassurance being issued. If an investigation 'just to make sure' is ordered, a very ambiguous message is given to the patient.

Symptom control is also important, not merely because symptoms are painful or unpleasant, but also as a strategy for reinforcing the position from which reassurance can be given.

Treatments principally comprise manipulation of the patient's diet, psychological therapies or drug treatments. In general practice the drug treatment is the usual, and perhaps the only, practical approach. The evidence on which to base detailed dietary manipulation, on the basis that food intolerance may be important, is still somewhat flimsy in general practice. Psychological therapies, although undoubtedly having a beneficial effect in selected patients, are not practical possibilities for many of us; the same can be said of hypnotherapy.

Controlled therapeutic trials in irritable bowel syndrome are difficult because of the large placebo response, the difficulties of setting objective measures of improvement, and the fluctuating nature of the condition. A recent review of drug therapy trials concluded that there was not a single published study that provided compelling evidence that any therapeutic agent is efficacious in the global treatment of irritable bowel syndrome. This is not to say that there is no treatment that is helpful, merely that none has been scientifically shown to be; it also may reflect poor sub-division of patients with diarrhoea-predominant and constipation-predominant irritable bowel syndrome, who may respond quite differently to the same therapeutic intervention.

As the pathophysiological basis of the syndrome is unclear, rational curative therapy is simply not possible. However, as there are no serious long-term sequelae or consequences to consider, symptomatic treatment would appear to be entirely appropriate. As the predominant symptom (for instance bloating, loose stools or pain) may differ between patients, treatment has to be tailored to the individual patient's needs.

The most commonly used treatments include bulking agents, anti-spasmodics, anti-diarrhoeals, tranquillizers, and antidepressants. The use of bran in particular is common. As might be expected it certainly can be shown to improve constipation, but it may make other symptoms, notably the incidence of pain, diarrhoea and urgency worse, particularly in patients who have irritable bowel syndrome characterized by pain and diarrhoea, rather than constipation. Many patients already have an adequate dietary intake of fibre, and blanket prescription of bran is not an appropriate therapeutic approach. The basis of successful treatment, leading to a reduction in symptom severity, is a careful history. If painful spasm predominates, then an anti-spasmodic is indicated; if diarrhoea predominates then an anti-diarrhoeal is indicated, and so on. It is, of course, important to explain that only symptomatic treatment is being attempted and that symptoms can be expected to recur in the future, but the demonstration that effective symptomatic relief is available is of considerable help in long-term management.

Elaborate dietary manipulations have been tried with some reports of success. However, a formal exclusion diet, on the basis of food intolerance, requires the expertise of a dietitian and is not a practical option for many patients. The elimination or reduction of caffeine intake has some anecdotal reports of benefit and has the merit of being largely achievable. Hypnotherapy and individual and group psychotherapy have all been reported as being helpful; interestingly, the effects of hypnotherapy sessions appear to have their beneficial action on visceral thresholds independent of their general pyschotherapeutic benefit. These are, however, not really practical options in general practice, although referral could be considered in some refractory cases and many gastroenterologists with a special interest in irritable bowel syndrome work closely with psychologists and psychiatrists in the out-patient clinic.

FURTHER READING

Crean, G. P. (1985). Towards a positive diagnosis of the irritable bowel syndrome. In *Irritable bowel syndrome* (ed. N. W. Read), pp. 29–41. Grune and Stratton, Florida.

Guthrie, E., Creed, F. H. and Whorwell, P. J. (1984). Severe sexual dysfunction in women with the irritable bowel syndrome: comparison with inflammatory bowel disease and duodenal ulceration. *British Medical Journal*, **285**, 577–8.

Guthrie, E. A., Creed, F. H., Whorwell, P. J. and Tomenson, B. (1992). Outpatients with irritable bowel syndrome: a comparison of first time and chronic attenders. *Gut*, **33**, 361–3.

Guthrie, E. and Creed, F. (1989). Psychological treatments of the irritable bowel syndrome: a review. *Gut*, **30**, 1601–9.

Heaton, K. W., Ghosh, S. and Braddon, F. E. M. (1991). How bad are the symptoms and bowel dysfunction of patients with irritable bowel syndrome? *Gut*, **32**, 73–9.

Holmes, K. M. and Salter, R. H. (1982). Irritable bowel syndrome—a safe diagnosis *British Medical Journal*, **285**, 1533–4.

Jones, R. and Lydeard, S. (1992). Irritable bowel syndrome in the general population. *British Medical Journal*, **304**, 87–90.

Kettell, J., Jones, R., and Lydeard, S. (1992). Reasons for consultation in irritable bowel syndrome: symptoms and patient characteristics. *British Journal of General Practice*, **42**, 459–61.

Manning, A. P., Thompson, W. G., Heaton, K. W. and Maris, A. I. (1978). Towards positive diagnosis of the irritable bowel. *British Medical Journal*, **2**, 653–4.

Talley, N. J., Phillips, S. F., Melton, L. J., Witgen, C. and Zinsmeister, A. K. (1989). A patient questionnaire to identify bowel disease. *Annals of Internal Medicine*, **11**, 671–4.

Talley, N. J., Phillips, S. F., Melton, L. J. and Zinsmeister, A. K. (1990). Diagnostic value of the Manning criteria in irritable bowel syndrome. *Gut*, **31**, 77–8.

Thompson, W. G., Doterall, G., Drossman, D. A., Heaton, K. W. and Kruis, W. (1989). Irritable bowel syndrome: guidelines for the diagnosis. *Gastroenterology International*, **2**, 92–5.

White, A. M., Stevens, W. H., Upton, A. R., O'Byrne, P. M. and Collins, S. M. (1991). Airway responsiveness to inhaled methacholine in patients with irritable bowel syndrome. *Gastroenterology*, **100**, 68–74.

9 Liver, biliary, and pancreatic problems

Ian Forgacs

In contrast to diseases of the 'hollow' gastrointestinal organs, diseases of the liver and pancreas are less usual in general practice. Clearly, the most common of the diseases within this group are those caused by gallstones but, even here, caution is needed before attributing a patient's symptoms to biliary calculi, since we recognize that several symptoms previously considered to be due to gallstones—such as fatty food intolerance—are not of biliary origin. Nevertheless, the presenting symptoms of acute hepato-biliary and pancreatic disease can be very striking and require careful initial evaluation. Early recognition that a problem might be due to chronic disease of these organs is also important. An accurate diagnosis needs careful clinical assessment and judicious selection of laboratory and radiological tests, but it is usually possible for a general practitioner to make substantial progress in diagnosis, although more sophisticated in-hospital investigation and treatment may prove necessary.

This chapter will discuss the most frequently encountered presentations of patients with acute and chronic liver disease, gallstones, biliary obstruction, and pancreatic problems. All of these can produce jaundice which, therefore, seems an ideal place to begin.

JAUNDICE

Jaundice is the result of an increased bilirubin concentration in the blood. Although hyperbilirubinaemia occurs when the plasma bilirubin level exceeds 17 mmol/l, jaundice only becomes apparent when the bilirubin concentration exceeds two to three times the upper limit of normal. Bilirubin is a pigment derived from the breakdown of haem, mainly from haemoglobin in red blood cells. In its lipid-soluble form, unconjugated bilirubin is transported to the liver, where it is conjugated (and thus made water soluble) before excretion into bile (Figure 9.1). In the fasting state, bilirubin is stored within the gall-bladder, where it mixes with the other constituents of bile, principally bile salts, cholesterol, and other lipids. In response to a meal, the gall-bladder contracts to deliver bile to the duodenum. Bilirubin in the intestine is metabolized to urobilinogen, most of which is excreted in stool (giving the motions their characteristic

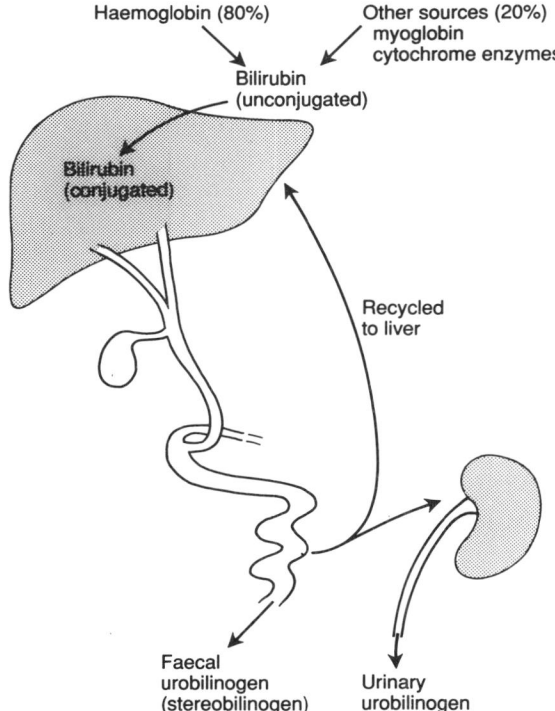

Haemoglobin (80%)

Other sources (20%)
myoglobin
cytochrome enzymes

Bilirubin
(unconjugated)

Bilirubin
(conjugated)

Recycled
to liver

Faecal
urobilinogen
(stereobilinogen)

Urinary
urobilinogen

Fig. 9.1 Bilirubin metabolism.

colour). A small proportion of urobilinogen is re-absorbed into portal blood and excreted by the kidneys. In health, therefore, bilirubin does not appear in the urine.

PRINCIPAL MECHANISMS OF JAUNDICE

Jaundice can be the result of physiological disturbance at a number of different sites in the metabolic pathway of bilirubin. It is essential to appreciate the main areas at which bilirubin metabolism can be disordered so as to understand the resultant differences between the various types of jaundice. Essentially, there are four different mechanisms (Table 9.1).

First, increased production of bilirubin may result from enhanced red cell breakdown, as seen in haemolytic anaemia. In this situation, the bilirubin in the blood is principally unconjugated and, unless haemolysis is severe, jaundice is usually mild. There will be an increase in the level of

Table 9.1 *Mechanisms and classification of jaundice*

Mechanisms
1. Increased bilirubin production.
2. Defective hepatic uptake of bilirubin.
3. Disturbed hepatic conjugation.
4. Disordered excretion of conjugated bilirubin.

Classification

Traditional	Contemporary
Pre-hepatic	Pre-hepatic
Hepatic	Hepatocellular
	Intrahepatic cholestasis
Post-hepatic	Extrahepatic cholestasis

---

urobilinogen in the urine, but not of bilirubin, so the jaundice is said to be acholuric.

Secondly, there may be a defect in the uptake of bilirubin by the liver. The most common cause of this is seen in Gilbert's syndrome, in which the synthetic and other detoxifying functions of the liver are quite normal. The hyperbilirubinaemia is unconjugated.

Thirdly, the process of conjugation by the liver can be disturbed. This is rare, occurs particularly in neonates, and will not be considered further here.

Fourthly, there may be a defect in the excretion of conjugated bilirubin. This may occur within the liver cell itself or at a site within the biliary tree as far distally as the duodenum. This is by far the most important mechanism in the production of jaundice in clinical practice, including as it does many diseases of the liver as well as obstructive jaundice due to gallstones or malignancy.

CLASSIFICATION OF JAUNDICE (TABLE 9.1)

There is still something to be said for the old-fashioned classification of jaundice into pre-hepatic, hepatic, and post-hepatic types. This classification is not, however, without its shortcomings. From the foregoing, it is readily appreciated that progress in our knowledge of how the body handles bilirubin means that there is a degree of overlap between them. While type 1 (above) is clearly pre-hepatic, type 4 importantly contains both hepatic and post-hepatic jaundice. It is more appropriate to consider pre-hepatic, hepatocellular, and cholestatic jaundice, the latter being defined as hyperbilirubinaemia where conjugated bilirubin fails to reach the duodenum. Thus, we can recognize cholestasis as a result of liver disease (intrahepatic) or because of obstruction to bile flow within the larger bile ducts (extrahepatic), and we can equate post-hepatic jaundice with the more modern term, extrahepatic cholestasis. In practice, liver diseases producing jaundice frequently involve both hepatocellular and cholestatic mechanisms.

COMMON CAUSES OF JAUNDICE IN CLINICAL PRACTICE (TABLE 9.2)

Gilbert's syndrome

This is the most common cause of an elevated level of unconjugated bilirubin and occurs in 2–4 per cent of the population. It is not of any functional significance and is usually recognized as an incidental finding on multi-channel biochemical analysis. Occasionally, patients may notice mild jaundice, particularly during periods of starvation or illness. This can lead to diagnostic confusion in the unwary. The blood count and other liver function tests are quite normal.

Haemolytic anaemia

When haemolysis is severe, jaundice may become apparent, although other clinical manifestations usually dominate the clinical picture. The level of unconjugated bilirubin is elevated and, in the urine, urobilinogen— but not bilirubin—is elevated (acholuric jaundice). The blood count will show anaemia with associated reticulocytosis.

Table 9.2 *Common causes of jaundice*

Pre-hepatic
Gilbert's syndrome
Haemolysis
Hepatocellular and intra-hepatic cholestasis
Acute viral hepatitis
Alcoholic hepatitis
Drug-induced jaundice
Chronic active hepatitis
Cirrhosis
Extra-hepatic cholestasis
Gallstones
Carcinoma of the pancreas

Viral hepatitis

This term includes infection not only by one of the recognized hepatitis viruses, A, B, and C, but also by one of the other viruses which can result in hepatitis as part of a wider systemic ilness. These include infectious mononucleosis due to Epstein–Barr virus and cytomegalovirus. In general, the clinical manifestations of viral hepatitis are similar whichever the causative agent, but there are important differences in their route of transmission and in their prognosis.

Hepatitis A

This infection is transmitted by the faecal-oral route. Epidemics may occur, but this form of hepatitis is often seen after foreign travel. The illness is usually mild and begins with a prodromal 'viral' illness before the onset of jaundice. It is uncommon for jaundice to last for more than three weeks but, rarely, cholestatic rather than hepatocellular jaundice can predominate and the patient may remain icteric for several months. Even when the infection resolves quickly, malaise can persist. Levels of transaminase enzymes, aspartate aminotransferase (AST), and alanine aminotransferase (ALT) in blood are high at the beginning of the illness, and IgM antibodies to hepatitis A virus are found in serum.

Hepatitis B

The main route of transmission is parenteral. Inoculation from contaminated blood transfusion has become much less common, but cases may occur in intravenous drug abusers from shared needles. In the UK, infection is most commonly seen in homosexuals. The incubation period is longer than for hepatitis A, and varies from three to six months, however clinical features and patterns of liver function tests are similar. Markers of hepatitis B virus are found in the blood, the hepatitis B surface antigen (HBsAg) appearing first, but levels of this antigen disappear within three months of the onset of jaundice and hepatitis B antibodies appear as the infection is eradicated. However, in some 5–10 per cent of cases, the infection can proceed into chronic hepatitis. It is important for patients to be followed up in the months following this infection to identify those with persistent hepatitis B antigenaemia who are at risk of developing chronic hepatitis, cirrhosis, and hepatocellular carcinoma.

Hepatitis C

Many of us have followed the nomenclature of hepatitis viruses with wry amusement. Non-A, non-B hepatitis was always a clumsy name, but with the identification of the hepatitis C virus is 1989, the term has become obsolescent. Hepatitis C is clinically similar to both of its alphabetical precursors but its route of transmission is similar to that of hepatitis B. It is most commonly seen in recipients of whole blood products, but may also be transmitted sexually. Although cases of hepatitis B in health workers have become less common since the introduction of effective vaccination, hepatitis C cannot, as yet, be prevented in this way. The diagnosis is made, to some extent, by the history of exposure and by exclusion of other viruses. There is a useful serological test for hepatitis C antibodies, but there are still some problems with the sensitivity and specificity of currently available tests. It seems that 50 per cent of cases of hepatitis C develop into a chronic phase.

Alcoholic hepatitis

Alcohol abuse can, of course, present in a myriad of ways in a variety of organ systems. Acute alcoholic hepatitis is one of its most striking manifestations. Jaundice is often rapidly progressive and may be associated with right upper quadrant abdominal pain and fever. Hepatitis may arise *de novo*, or may complicate pre-existing recognized alcoholic liver disease. An alcohol history should always be vigorously sought. Laboratory values are not diagnostic of the underlying cause but marked elevation of transaminases and the gamma-glutamyl transpeptidase (gamma GT) are typical, and the level of bilirubin may be very high. A raised erythrocyte mean cell volume is suggestive of, but not specific for, alcoholism. This condition should be treated in hospital as the mortality may exceed 30 per cent. Some cases respond to corticosteroid therapy.

Drug jaundice

The range of effects that drugs may have on the liver is enormous, and may range from innocuous elevations of liver enzymes by induction (for example, anti-convulsants) to life-threatening hepatocellular damage (for example, paracetamol overdose). Drugs can cause jaundice by interference with bilirubin metabolism, by causing direct hepatotoxicity, by hypersensitivity, and by cholestasis. Some 10 per cent of cases of jaundice seen in specialized units, such as King's College Hospital, London, are attributable to drug toxicity. Some of the more commonly implicated drugs are listed in Table 9.3.

Proof that a drug is responsible for jaundice may be impossible, as it can be difficult to exclude coincident viral hepatitis. Nevertheless, it is most important to consider drug therapy as a cause of jaundice in every case. Usually, the jaundice will subside on stopping the drug and it is, of course, vital that a practitioner recognizes the association to avoid a repeat prescription.

Table 9.3 *Commonly implicated drugs in jaundice*

Antibiotics
Sulphonamides
Erythromycin
Tetracyclines

Anti-tuberculous agents
Isoniazid
Rifampicin
Pyrazinamide

Psychotrophic drugs
Phenothiazines, particularly chlorpromazine
Mono-amine oxidase inhibitors
Tri-cyclic antidepressants

Steroid hormones
Androgens
Oestrogens
Progestogens

Anaesthetics
Halothane

Cytotoxics
Methotrexate
Azathioprine

Anti-hypertensives
Methyldopa
Thiazides

Chronic active hepatitis and cirrhosis

While these conditions can present insidiously, the onset of jaundice may
be an initial manifestation, therefore chronic liver disease should be
considered in any patient presenting with jaundice. Chronic hepatitis and
cirrhosis are discussed in more detail below, but it is appropriate to
consider here some of the clues that might indicate that a jaundiced patient
may have a chronic disease. There may, of course, be an antecedent
history of liver disease, but physical signs can be especially helpful. Palmar
erythema, leuconychia, clubbing, Dupuytren's contracture, spider naevi,
and gynaecomastia are all readily detectable, but are not invariable.
Hepatomegaly and/or splenomegaly are also variable, the presence of an

enlarged spleen may be an indicator of portal hypertension, although splenomegaly can occur acutely in viral hepatitis. Portal hypertension may give rise to shifting dullness characteristic of ascites. Ultimately, the diagnosis will rest on more sophisticated laboratory and histological evaluation.

Extrahepatic obstruction

Cholestatic jaundice is the most common presenting feature of extrahepatic obstruction and, although there is a variety of inflammatory and infiltrating diseases which narrow the biliary tree, the two most frequently seen are gallstones and carcinoma of the head of the pancreas. A careful history is most helpful. There may be evidence of previous episodes of biliary colic, and patients with carcinoma of the ampulla of Vater or pancreas may also notice upper abdominal pain that radiates to the back, but such a history is by no means the rule. Patients with obstructive jaundice will have pale stools and dark urine that contains bilirubin but not urobilinogen. Pruritus, which may be intense, is a useful pointer. The liver is often enlarged, and a palpably distended gall-bladder is very suggestive of a neoplastic stricture (Courvoisier's law). Biochemically, the level of alkaline phosphatase is usually very high, relatively much more than the modest rise seen in the level of transaminases. The key investigation is an ultrasound scan which, in obstructive jaundice, will show a dilated bilary tree, although it is less usual for the radiologist to identify the actual site of obstruction. Stones in the common bile duct are often not visualized, neither are pancreatic tumours, unless they are quite large (> 5 cm).

A DIAGNOSTIC APPROACH TO JAUNDICE

The initial steps in the clinical evaluation and investigation of a jaundiced patient are listed in Table 9.4.

Social history

Occupational hazards should be noted. In particular, whether alcohol exposure is likely, or whether there might be contact with rats suggesting leptospirosis (Weil's disease).

Possible contacts with jaundice may be relevant, particularly in closed environments. A history of sexual behaviour is helpful in the diagnosis of hepatitis B and C. Patients should be asked if they have had any injections or transfusions within the preceding six months.

Recent foreign travel or an ethnic origin from the Mediterranean area, Africa, or the Far East may suggest specific types of viral hepatitis.

Table 9.4 *Steps in clinical evaluation and investigation of jaundice*

History
Social
   Occupation
   Contacts
   Sexual behaviour
   Injections/transfusions
   Travel
Drugs
Alcohol
Past history
   Surgery
   Previous post-operative jaundice
Gastro-intestinal symptoms
   Bowel habit
   Abdominal pain
   Anorexia/weight loss
Antecedent symptoms

Examination
Physical (see Fig. 9.2)
Urine/stool

Laboratory
Liver function tests
   Bilirubin
   Alkaline phosphatase
   Gammaglutamyl transpeptidase
   Transaminases (ALT, AST)
   Plasma proteins
      albumin
      globulin
Haematology
   Blood count
   Prothrombin time
Serology
   Viral markers—hepatitis A, B and C
   Paul-Bunnell test
   Cytomegalovirus antibodies

Radiology
Ultrasound
ERCP

Drugs

Patients should be closely questioned about any drug treatment. The author's experience in hospital practice is that many patients are unsure of their medication.

Alcohol

A high index of suspicion is necessary. Information from a relative may be helpful. Such symptoms as morning nausea and anorexia are common in those drinking sufficient to have serious liver toxicity.

Past medical history

Previous biliary surgery raises the possibility of residual/recurrent common duct stones or bile duct stricture. A history of malignant disease raises the possibility of hepatic metastases. Post-operative jaundice may implicate halothane as a cause.

Gastrointestinal symptoms

The combination of pale stools, dark urine, and pruritus suggests bile duct obstruction. Previous episodes of biliary colic suggest gallstones as the cause of the obstruction. In pancreatic cancer, jaundice may be painless, but progressive anorexia, weight loss, and pain radiating to the back can occur.

Antecedent symptoms

Prodromal 'flu-like' symptoms in the week before jaundice rapidly appears suggests viral hepatitis, as do nausea, anorexia, and an aversion to smoking. The onset of jaundice is usually within just a few hours in viral hepatitis, and is more rapid than in other hepatic or obstructive biliary diseases. High fever and rigors typify acute cholangitis.

EXAMINATION

Many of the physical signs that might be relevant to the diagnosis of jaundice are illustrated in Fig. 9.2.

General findings

The degree and tinge of jaundice may reflect the underlying pathology. In pre-hepatic conditions, jaundice is of a mild yellow hue. In hepatocellular

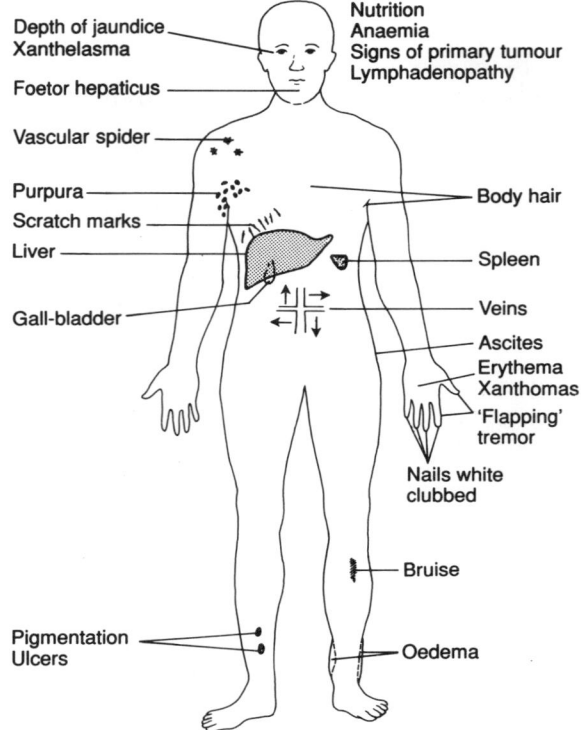

Fig. 9.2 Physical signs in jaundice.

disease the colour is more orange, while in extra-hepatic obstruction, the discerning observer can detect a dark greenish tinge.

Anaemia accompanies haemolysis and may be seen in cirrhosis.

Obvious weight loss is non-specific but suggests cancer or advanced cirrhosis.

Skin changes include bruising (when a coagulopathy complicates cirrhosis) and scratch-marks (when cholestatic disease causes pruritus).

Abdominal examination

The key features are shown in Fig. 9.2. Hepatomegaly is a very non-specific finding, but a large, nodular liver is suspicious of neoplasia. Splenomegaly is found in chronic, and occasionally also acute, liver disease but may be a feature of haemolytic anaemia.

Urine and faecal examination

Bilirubin in the urine is an early feature of viral hepatitis. Absence of urinary urobilinogen suggests complete biliary obstruction, while increased levels (in the absence of bilirubin) indicate haemolysis. Pale stools indicate biliary obstruction.

Laboratory investigations

These should include, as initial investigations in all jaundiced patients, biochemical tests and haematology.

Biochemical tests (liver function tests)

Serum bilirubin

This will confirm jaundice, and serial testing is useful in following the progress of the condition. In practice, it is rarely necessary to ask the laboratory to measure separately the unconjugated and conjugated fractions.

Serum alkaline phosphatase

This enzyme is not specific for the liver but is found in a number of other tissues, mainly bone. If the origin of an elevated level is unclear, an accompanying rise in gamma GT indicates a hepatobiliary origin. The alkaline phosphatase is most significantly elevated in cholestatic jaundice (usually at least three times normal) and less so in hepatocellular disease. High levels can be seen in malignant infiltration.

Serum transaminases

The alanine aminotransferase is more specific for liver disease than the aspartate aminotransferase (which is also found in cardiac and skeletal muscle), although the tissue responsible for elevating the enzyme level is rarely in doubt. Levels are highest when jaundice is hepatocellular (especially in hepatitis) with less marked increases in cholestasis. Transaminases are markers of liver inflammation and fall rapidly as hepatic injury lessens—either spontaneously in viral hepatitis or with treatment in chronic liver disease.

Plasma proteins

The total protein and albumin (and by inference total globulin) levels are usually normal at the onset of jaundice unless there is chronic liver disease, when the albumin level may be low. An elevated globulin level may be seen in immunologically-mediated liver disease.

Interpretation of liver function tests

A note of caution is needed for those who seek to find too much information in liver function tests. They are not true tests of liver function, but are biochemical variables which can reflect a range of insults to the liver. As we have seen above, there are typical patterns in different types of insult to the liver but no test result (or pattern of results) is specific to a particular condition (or even to a group of conditions). They are an aid to diagnosis and a guide to progression of the disease, but it is an unwise physician indeed whose clinical diagnosis rests mainly on the results of these tests.

Haematological tests

The combination of anaemia and reticulocytosis suggests haemolysis and the need for further haematological work-up. Changes in the blood, such as leucocytosis, are not otherwise likely to be specific for diagnosing the cause of jaundice, although they can act as a guide. A prolonged prothrombin time that corrects after vitamin K injection indicates cholestasis, while failure to correct suggests hepatocellular disease.

Serological tests

If infectious hepatitis is suspected, a search for viral markers must be undertaken. Hepatitis A IgM antibody and hepatitis B surface antigen screening are readily available. All patients with jaundice in whom hepatitis B is a remote possibility should be screened. The limitations of present tests for hepatitis C antibodies have already been mentioned. The Paul-Bunnell test and cytomegalovirus antibody testing might also be appropriate. A patient with a hepatitis-like illness but negative virology should be referred to hospital.

Radiological investigation

Conventional radiology in the presence of jaundice was either difficult or more usually impossible because of the failure of the liver to excrete contrast media. However, ultrasound scanning is able to answer the critical question of whether, in the presence of cholestatic jaundice, there is extrahepatic obstruction. If dilated bile ducts are seen, there is a need for prompt referral for further imaging to define the precise site of obstruction, which is most appropriately done by endoscopic retrograde cholangio-pancreatography (ERCP). The major advantage of ERCP over other radiological imaging techniques in this situation is that an indwelling stent can be passed endoscopically into the bile duct to decompress the obstruction.

CHRONIC LIVER DISEASE

These conditions tend to present insidiously and they often produce non-specific symptoms so that recognition depends on having a high index of clinical suspicion. The more common forms of chronic liver disease are listed in Table 9.5.

CHRONIC ACTIVE HEPATITIS

This is a syndrome in which several different aetiologies result in a similar picture, both in terms of the resulting liver damage and their clinical features. The most common form in the UK is auto-immune chronic active hepatitis (which is 2–3 times more frequent in women), but in parts of the world where the infection is endemic, chronic hepatitis B infection is a major health problem (which is ten times more common in men). We have already discussed how both hepatitis B and C can persist after the acute infective episode.

Clinical features

About one third of patients with the auto-immune form of the disease present with a hepatitis-like illness, which may seem to resolve only to reappear. The remainder, and most of those with chronic viral infection, tend to have more non-specific symptoms, such as general malaise. Occasionally, multi-organ symptoms typical of systemic auto-immune disease, such as joint pains, fever, and haemolytic anaemia occur. Many patients already have established cirrhosis at the time of diagnosis.

Table 9.5 *Common forms of chronic liver disease*

Chronic active hepatitis
Autoimmune
Viral hepatitis—B and C

Cirrhosis
Alcoholic
Chronic active hepatitis
Metabolic
    Haemochromatosis
    Wilson's disease
Primary biliary cirrhosis

Examination can be quite normal, but it may reveal the stigmata of chronic liver disease. However, clinical assessment alone is insufficient to indicate the aetiology and it is critical to make a precise diagnosis as specific treatment is available.

Investigation

Liver function tests usually show a hepatitic picture with elevation of the transaminases. In the auto-immune form, the globulin fraction of proteins is typically raised and immunological abnormalities are present as a high titre of antinuclear factor (ANF) and anti-smooth muscle antibodies are found. These immunological tests are normal in chronic viral infection but serology will show markers of persisting hepatitis B infection. Referral to hospital for liver biopsy is mandatory.

Treatment

The auto-immune form of chronic active hepatitis responds well to corticosteroids, initially in high dose. Long-term treatment is usually necessary and the dosage of prednisolone is tailored to maintain liver function tests within the normal range. Often, azathioprine is added as an adjunct to allow a lower dose of steroids to be used. Corticosteroids are contra-indicated in chronic active hepatitis B and C for which, hitherto, there has been no effective therapy. However, quite recently, the anti-viral agent, interferon, has been shown to be effective in about 30–40 per cent of patients in a number of clinical trials.

CIRRHOSIS

Cirrhosis is, by contrast, an irreversible condition characterized by fibrosis and regenerative nodules within the liver. It is the end-result of a variety of conditions, which include alcoholic liver disease, chronic active hepatitis, and primary biliary cirrhosis. Less commonly, metabolic diseases, such as haemochromatosis and Wilson's disease lead to cirrhosis as a result, respectively, of iron and copper deposition in the liver.

Clinical features

Although patients with cirrhosis may have been recognized to have an antecedent liver condition if they have presented in some of the ways we have already discussed, it is not uncommon for presentation of cirrhosis to be delayed until complications develop. The two most important such complications are portal hypertension and liver cell failure.

Portal hypertension presents either as abdominal distension due to ascites or as gastrointestinal bleeding from oesophageal varices. Chronic liver failure produces the syndrome of hepatic encephalopathy which gives rise to a clinical spectrum ranging from impaired judgement and mild confusion to a more profound impairment of consciousness and, ultimately, coma. The syndrome often follows precipitants, such as infection, electrolyte disturbance (especially after enthusiastic diuretic use) or gastrointestinal bleeding. The development of encephalopathy implies advanced liver disease and consequently a poor prognosis. A flapping tremor of the outstretched, extended hands is a useful physical sign.

Investigation

The diagnosis of cirrhosis can be obvious when, for example, an alcoholic with advanced disease presents with all the cutaneous signs of chronic liver disease accompanied by ascites. Investigations show deranged liver function tests, often with a low albumin and prolonged prothrombin time due to reduced protein synthesis by the liver. The diagnosis should be confirmed by liver biopsy if possible. A search will be made in hospital for potentially treatable conditions, especially in the younger patient when there is a possibility of a metabolic disease. Like chronic active hepatitis, primary biliary cirrhosis may be detected at a pre-cirrhotic stage. This slowly progressive condition is found mostly in middle-aged women. The brunt of liver injury is borne by the bile ducts and this diagnosis may be suspected when the alkaline phosphatase and gamma GT levels are found to be elevated on screening biochemistry. There is a characteristic immunological abnormality of anti-mitochondrial antibodies in serum. Hyperlipidaemia is common, leading to skin xanthomas, and pruritus may be a particularly distressing symptom.

Treatment

There is no specific treatment for cirrhosis, but underlying treatable conditions, such as chronic active hepatitis, should be identified so that therapy may halt disease progression. It is absolutely crucial that patients with alcoholic cirrhosis abstain from alcohol as this substantially improves their prognosis. There is, as yet, no definitely established treatment for primary biliary cirrhosis.

Nutritional advice is helpful, especially in malnourished alcoholics. However, those with encephalopathy should have a low-protein diet. Restrictions on salt and fluid intake may inhibit formation of ascites, but the mainstay of treatment here are diuretics. Spironolactone is the drug of choice. The onset of gastrointestinal bleeding clearly necessitates hospital admission and this is usually also necessary in those who develop ascites or encephalopathy. Pioneering work in Cambridge and London has firmly established liver transplantation as a therapeutic option and this should certainly be considered in patients with end-stage disease.

GALLSTONES

The time-honoured adage that the typical patient with gallstones is fair, fat, fertile, and forty does not wholly stand up to epidemiological investigation. It is true that obesity, parity, and the female sex are risk factors, but the incidence of gallstones rises with increasing age in both sexes. The majority of gallstones are composed predominantly of cholesterol, although 10 per cent contain mainly calcium salts. Cholesterol is held in solution by the other lipid components of bile, but when the balance between them is disturbed, cholesterol precipitates initially as crystals from which calculi later grow.

The majority of patients with gallstones are asymptomatic, but stones can give rise to a number of clinical conditions listed in Table 9.6. Biliary colic is the most common presenting symptom. This is usually a constant (rather than colicky pain) in the epigastrium or right hypochondrium which may be severe, often lasts for several hours and is accompanied by vomiting. Its aetiology is still somewhat unclear, but is believed to be due to transient impaction of small stones within the extra-hepatic biliary tree. Acute cholecystitis should not be confused with biliary colic. Here, there is inflammation of the gall-bladder resulting in right-sided upper abdominal pain which may radiate to the shoulder together with fever and marked local tenderness. Obstructive jaundice follows impaction of a stone in the common bile duct. Cholangitis may develop if infection occurs above the obstruction giving rise to the classical triad of fever, rigors, and jaundice. If a stone impacts within the ampulla of Vater, acute pancreatitis may develop (this is discussed below). Finally, carcinoma of the gall-bladder is an unusual tumour but is certainly very uncommon in the absence of gallstones. This usually presents with jaundice, which may be painless, although right-sided abdominal pain may be a feature.

Table 9.6 *Clinical conditions related to gallstones*

Biliary colic
Acute cholecystitis
Obstructive jaundice
Acute cholangitis
Acute pancreatitis
Carcinoma of the gall-bladder

Gallstones are not a cause of dyspepsia nor of fatty food intolerance but may be found incidentally during investigation of such symptoms. This has become a more common occurrence since ultrasound scanning has become widely available. Several long-term follow-up studies of patients who have been incidentally found to have gallstones have established that such stones usually remain asymptomatic. It is clear that the gallstones (and gall-bladders) of such patients should be left well alone, unless symptoms develop. The clinician should make every effort to decide whether to incriminate gallstones as the cause of symptoms and there is no substitute for a careful clinical evaluation.

Investigation

Most gallstones are radiolucent so are not seen on plain X-rays. However, ultrasound has largely replaced oral cholecystography in the diagnosis of gallstones. The development of acute complications, such as cholecystitis, jaundice, suspected cholangitis, and pancreatitis are indications for referral to hospital.

Treatment

Therapy of gallstone disease has undergone a revolution over the past 20 years. Conventional cholecystectomy has been challenged successively by oral bile acid treatment (of limited application and with disappointing long-term results, as stones often return even after successful dissolution) and shock-wave lithotripsy (which is very expensive and, again, stones may return). A variety of other ingenious, technically-demanding, non-operative interventions have been developed but without wide acceptance. The recent development of laparoscopic cholecystectomy has, however, gained favour both among surgeons (who, doubtless, enjoy the challenge of learning new techniques) and patients, who are attracted to short hospital stays (perhaps a couple of days, or even less) and the avoidance of anything other than a small incision and the associated discomfort of the conventional operation.

Bile duct obstruction is also best detected by ultrasound, although when stones are impacted, they often cannot be identified. The site and nature of the obstructing lesion is best diagnosed by ERCP. The endoscopist has a role not only in diagnosis but in treatment of biliary obstruction. Common bile duct stones are now usually treated endoscopically. This technique has major advantages over surgery, particularly for those for whom biliary surgery carries a real mortality—the jaundiced, the elderly, and those with cardiac, respiratory or other medical conditions.

PANCREATIC DISEASES

In clinical practice, the three most important conditions are acute and chronic pancreatitis and pancreatic cancer.

ACUTE PANCREATITIS

The most common aetiological factors are alcohol abuse, especially following a binge in a habitually heavy drinker, and gallstones. Mild attacks may result from viral infection and some cases are idiopathic. Acute pancreatitis presents as acute, severe, upper abdominal pain. It is usually of fairly sudden onset and the pain may radiate to the back and be accompanied by vomiting. The differential diagnosis is that of any cause of the acute abdomen, particularly perforation of a peptic ulcer. On examination, the patient may obviously be in severe discomfort with abdominal rigidity, tenderness, and guarding. Tachycardia and hypotension may be apparent and shock can occur in severe cases. The diagnosis is confirmed by an elevated serum amylase level and the condition should always be treated in hospital as the overall mortality is at least 10 per cent.

CHRONIC PANCREATITIS

This results from inflammation of the pancreas which eventually leads to fibrosis and consequent destruction of pancreatic glandular tissue. In about half of the cases, no aetiological factor can be identified but the most commonly identified cause is chronic alcoholism. Other factors include congenital abnormalities of pancreatic structure and metabolic disturbances such as some forms of hyperlipidaemia and hypercalcaemia. The principal symptom is chronic upper abdominal pain, radiating to the back. This is often very severe and continuous, but may be eased by leaning forward. Eating may aggravate the pain so that anorexia is common. Nausea and vomiting may occur. Symptoms of pancreatic enzyme deficiency may lead to steatorrhoea which aggravates the tendency for these patients to lose weight. This condition is best investigated by a specialist. The diagnosis is made by finding evidence of structural damage (calcified pancreas on plain X-ray, ultrasound, CT scan or ERCP—in ascending order of diagnostic yield), or functional deficiency (steatorrhoea and evidence of pancreatic exocrine dysfunction by tubed or tubeless pancreatic function tests). The serum amylase level has no value in the diagnosis of chronic pancreatitis. Treatment is supportive. Alcohol abstinence is crucial. Analgesics, possibly opiates, and nutritional support, with pancreatic enzyme supplements are the mainstays of treatment in what is often a very chronic and long-lasting illness.

CARCINOMA OF THE PANCREAS

This is the third most common gastrointestinal malignancy (after colorectal and stomach cancer) with 5500 new cases each year in England and Wales. The incidence is rising, but the reason for this is not known as the aetiology is quite unclear. The condition is more common in smokers, but not, as was once thought, in coffee drinkers or alcoholics. There may be an increased incidence in chronic pancreatitis. Symptoms tend to occur late and are often non-specific. Weight loss is usual and may be accompanied by abdominal pain. Jaundice implies bile duct obstruction. Vomiting may result from duodenal or gastric obstruction and diarrhoea and steatorrhoea can occur. In addition to the patient appearing unwell with obvious signs of weight loss, examination may reveal an abdominal mass, hepatomegaly or jaundice (perhaps with a palpable gall-bladder). Laboratory tests are not specific, but anaemia and a high erythrocyte sedimentation rate are common. Liver function tests may suggest extrahepatic obstruction or secondary spread. Ultrasound sometimes identifies a pancreatic mass, but a negative scan very definitely does not exclude this diagnosis. If pancreatic carcinoma is suspected, hospital referral should be made. CT scanning and ERCP are superior to ultrasound in this situation. A tissue diagnosis should be made and it is usually possible to manage patients with pancreatic cancer without surgery unless there are real prospects of operative resectability (in perhaps 10 per cent of patients), or palliation cannot be achieved by non-surgical means. Few patients survive one year from the time of diagnosis.

10 Rectal bleeding and lower bowel problems

Jeremy Barnes and Michael Farthing

The passage of recognizable blood per rectum is a common cause of great concern to many patients, who will hurry along to their doctor for advice and reassurance. By contrast, there is a much larger group of patients who make the same observation and who react in a contrary way and do not present to their doctor at all. Rectal bleeding is an important symptom which should never be dismissed lightly by the patient's doctor.

PREVALENCE AND NATURE OF RECTAL BLEEDING

Several studies have demonstrated that rectal bleeding is extremely common in the community and the prevalence of rectal bleeding is estimated at 12–16 per cent per year, although only a small but unrecorded proportion of these people will consult their doctor because of their bleeding. Blood may be noticed on the toilet paper, in the lavatory pan water, dripping or squirting from the anus, or be described as being mixed intimately with the stool. A further group of patients will report bloody diarrhoea.

The nature of the blood loss is a highly significant predictor for important colorectal disease. A quarter of those patients describing dark blood mixed in with their stool will have an important cause for their bleeding, while only 3 per cent of those reporting loss of bright-red blood will be found to have an important disorder. It is therefore crucial that we take a detailed history of the nature of the blood loss, as this is the single most helpful symptom that can indicate serious disease. This becomes ever more relevant with increase in the patient's age, since colorectal cancer (nearly 24 000 new cases annually in the UK) becomes increasingly common in each decade over the age of 40 years.

RECTAL BLEEDING NOT ASSOCIATED WITH DIARRHOEA

Torrential bleeding

Torrential blood loss is rare and is always recognizable as blood, however high up the bowel its origin. Most heavy bleeding with frank blood being passed per rectum comes from gastric or duodenal ulceration or oesophageal varices, although, more rarely, bleeding may occur from the small bowel, a Meckel's diverticulum, or from the colon.

Melaena

A slower loss from higher up the bowel may have time to undergo partial digestion and so will be passed as typical black tarry melaena stools with their characteristic odour. Melaena usually arises from a lesion in the oesophagus, stomach or duodenum.

Red blood mixed in with the stool

Blood mixed in with the stool is a highly significant observation suggestive of more proximal colonic disease, usually a carcinoma. Such bleeding is often dark in colour; it should never be attributed to haemorrhoids without a careful investigation of the lower bowel.

Red blood loss per rectum not mixed in with the stool

This usually originates from the lower colon, rectum, or anus. In general, the brighter the blood the lower the source. Heavier red blood loss may originate higher up the bowel, being passed so swiftly that it does not have time to alter in colour. By contrast, bright-red blood dripping from the anus at defecation will be from the anal canal and usually originates from the anal cushions or haemorrhoids. Bleeding from haemorrhoids may be associated with some anal discomfort, while a lesser blood loss accompanied by considerable pain suggests the presence of an anal fissure. Patients may also report small quantities of bright-red blood loss on the toilet paper as a result of over-zealous cleansing of the perianal area after defecation with consequent excoriation.

Bloody diarrhoea

This may be acute or chronic. Bloody diarrhoea of a few days duration is most likely to be infective in origin and enquiry should be made concerning recent foreign travel, and also about other affected contacts. It is important to enquire about the patient's occupation, and to be aware of the need to isolate a patient with possible infective diarrhoea whose job involves handling food. Doctors also have a statutory duty to notify the local Environmental Health Department of cases of *suspected* food poisoning and certain confirmed infections.

More long-standing bloody diarrhoea is likely to be due to some form of inflammatory bowel disease, usually ulcerative colitis, Crohn's colitis, or non-specific proctitis.

While inflammatory bowel disease may present at any age, the peak incidence occurs in the young adult.

It is clear that a detailed history of bowel function and of the nature of blood loss per rectum is essential in order to establish a cause or causes for the patient's symptoms. We need further information, for example, as to the duration of symptoms, the presence or absence of pain or discomfort, tenesmus, and whether the patient is passing mucus. Only with this information can we approach the investigation of the patient in a structured way.

As general practitioners we have to weigh up the relative risks for the patients. On the one hand we may treat obvious disorders such as haemorrhoids in the young without further investigation of the bowel, while, on the other hand, we must be aware that other important conditions may coexist with such obvious disorders, particularly in the older patient. This coexistence has been amply demonstrated by an Australian study of 145 patients over the age of 40 years with a history of less than six months' rectal bleeding. There was a high prevalence (63 per cent) of haemorrhoids concurrent with colonic lesions and 114 out of their 145 patients had haemorrhoids. However, they also concluded that the patient's description of their rectal bleeding was not helpful in differentiating anal from colorectal disease.

Occult blood loss

Occult bleeding is common and may be the only discernable sign of an important lesion, typically a carcinoma of the right side of the colon or caecum, when it may be accompanied by a persisting iron deficiency anaemia. Occult blood loss may also be a sign of blood loss from colonic polyps or early carcinoma. The screening of asymptomatic patients in general practice by faecal occult blood screening is dealt with in Chapter 11.

INVESTIGATION OF THE PATIENT WITH RECTAL BLEEDING

General physical examination may detect weight loss, anaemia or jaundice, and abdominal examination may reveal areas of tenderness, an abdominal mass or hepatomegaly. It is worth emphasizing that all patients with a history of blood loss per rectum must receive a careful rectal examination. This may seem to be obvious, but unfortunately there is evidence that this is not always carried out in general practice.

Bleeding from the perianal area

Examination of the anus may reveal eczematization of the perianal skin or painful fissuring, both of which may bleed slightly as a result of abrasion by toilet paper.

Haemorrhoids or piles

Thrombosed perianal vein (perianal haematoma or external pile)

The sudden development of a painful and tender swelling at one point in the perianal area is due to thrombosis of a perianal vein, perhaps caused by a period of straining at stool. It is unfortunately named and has nothing to do with piles and is not a haematoma. Such acute lesions may burst discharging altered blood and causing considerable alarm. Distinction from true haemorrhoids is not difficult, since a thrombosed perianal vein is covered by true skin.

True haemorrhoids

True haemorrhoids are formed as a result of the stretching, congestion, and disruption of the anal cushions, often associated with long-standing constipation and straining at stool. They may eventually prolapse through the anus and so be visible externally. They can be distinguished from a thrombosed perianal vein by their mucosal covering which may cause a mucoid discharge. By asking the patient to strain it may be possible to demonstrate prolapsing haemorrhoids.

Haemorrhoids are divided into three categories, first-degree where there is enlargement of the anal cushions, second-degree where there is prolapse of a part of the cushion on straining at stool which replaces itself, and third-degree where there is extensive prolapse of haemorrhoids at defecation which has to be replaced manually. About 50% per cent of people over the age of 50 years have haemorroids.

Digital rectal examination

This is a valuable procedure which must be carried out—indeed it is negligent to ignore it. A recent survey of rectal examination carried out in general practice revealed that fewer rectal examinations are carried out in smaller practices and in urban practices, and the decision to perform the examination was greatly influenced by patient's and doctor's gender and also a reluctance to cause embarrassment. The factors are not relevant to establishing the cause of a patient's blood loss and may seriously delay the diagnosis of serious disease.

The examining finger can usually reach about 8 cm from the anus and will be able to feel the whole circumference of the lower rectum and anal canal. It is usually not possible to feel haemorrhoids unless thrombosis has occurred—when the procedure is likely to be painful. In addition, rectal examination may also be very painful or actually not possible due to pain in the presence of an anal fissure. This may cause slight bleeding and usually is accompanied by an obvious skin tag, the so-called 'sentinel pile' external to the anus. Such fissures are accompanied by considerable sphincter spasm, which is usually absent with chronic fissures associated with Crohn's disease. The application of lignocaine (2 per cent) into the anal canal for a few minutes can ease the patient's discomfort considerably, making examination possible. Digital rectal examination can reach 15 per cent of colorectal tumours, most rectal carcinomas, and many adenomatous rectal polyps.

Proctoscopy

This is a simple, safe, and easy procedure which complements digital examination. It is possible to view the lower rectal mucosa which may show evidence of inflammatory change with loss of the normal vascular pattern, as in ulcerative colitis or the presence of multiple small ulcers as in Crohn's colitis. Polyps or carcinoma may also be seen occasionally. Haemorrhoids are obvious as folds of congested anal cushions involving the whole circumference just above the pectinate line. If proctoscopy is performed immediately, a bleeding point can often be seen. Asking the patient to strain to push out the instrument will give an idea of the extent of the haemorrhoids.

Rigid sigmoidoscopy

Rigid sigmoidoscopy is a misnomer and does not adequately examine the sigmoid. It is in reality a means of examining and, where necessary, taking biopsies from the rectum. Often it is possible to reach and sometimes look around the rectosigmoid junction. This is an area that contrast barium X-rays may not view adequately and so these investigations are complementary.

This procedure is one which can be satisfactorily performed in general practice. It requires no preparation, sedation or aftercare and is very safe and well-tolerated. Like any other skill it requires an initial period of training and practice. Many general practitioners will already be experienced at sigmoidoscopy as a result of their hospital-based training. Where necessary, teaching can usually be arranged with a local consultant gastroenterologist at his or her out-patient clinic. It is necessary to maintain such skills, and so it is sensible for one nominated partner to carry out all of the practice sigmoidoscopies. It is likely that a doctor with an average list of patients will request about two sigmoidoscopies per month for his or her symptomatic patients, although like any other procedure it will be used more if it is readily available. The cost of suitable equipment is considered later in this chapter.

Where 'in-practice' examination is not available then it is necessary to refer patients with rectal bleeding for investigation, either to an open-access sigmoidoscopy clinic if one is available, or to a hospital out-patient clinic. In some district hospitals sigmoidoscopy is required before a referral for barium enema examination will be accepted.

Flexible fibre-optic sigmoidoscopy

Flexible sigmoidoscopy employs a 60 cm fibre-optic instrument which can provide excellent views of the lower bowel up into the descending colon, and in many patients up to the splenic flexure. The examination is carried out after bowel preparation either using sodium picosulphate (Picolax) taken orally the day before the procedure, or an enema administered just before the examination. Flexible sigmoidoscopy is a safe and well-tolerated procedure which does not normally cause sufficient discomfort to require sedation, in addition biopsies can be taken at the time of the examination. It is thus a very suitable procedure to be carried out in primary care, and already several practices in the UK are performing flexible sigmoidoscopy, either in their practice or at adjacent general practitioner hospitals. At present the capital cost of setting up such a service is considerable, but in the context of fund-holding practices the use of a fibre-optic sigmoidoscope makes economic as well as clinical sense.

Referral

Where examination in the practice does not reveal a cause for the patient's rectal bleeding then referral for further investigation is essential. There are two avenues of investigation possible—sigmoidoscopy followed by barium enema, or colonoscopy—and the choice depends largely on the facilities available at the local district general hospital.

Some districts provide a general practice referral open-access sigmoido-scopy service such as that provided at Gloucester. Patients at this clinic are initially examined using a rigid instrument without bowel preparation; if a cause for bleeding is not found then a phosphate enema is given and the examination is repeated using a flexible sigmoidoscope. A written report is then sent to the patient's general practitioner who retains clinical responsibility for the patient.

Where flexible sigmoidoscopy is not available, double contrast barium enema X-ray is used to examine the bowel to the caecum after prior rigid sigmoidoscopy. Unfortunately, many district general hospitals do not offer access to their general practitioners to refer their patients for barium enema and so all such patients require referral to out-patients—an expensive use of medical manpower often involving unacceptable delay.

Even in skilled hands, air contrast barium enema examination is not as effective as colonoscopy during which the endoscopist may take tissue samples and remove polypoid lesions using diathermy. In spite of its undoubted benefits, colonoscopy is expensive, time-consuming, and less pleasant for the patient, who requires sedation and sometimes analgesia. In most districts because of limited facilities it is used selectively for the problem patient, in whom full investigation has not provided a diagnosis. By contrast a number of centres offer open access colonoscopy to their local general practitioners. One such service in Southampton reported a 57 per cent yield of significant disease, with 14 patients found to have colorectal cancer out of 137 referrals by the general practitioner.

In the ideal situation there is no doubt that colonoscopy is the investigation of choice for the patient with unexplained blood loss from the bowel.

A PRACTICAL APPROACH TO MANAGEMENT

Although there are variations in facilities, both between practices and between health districts, it is still possible to take a structured approach to the investigation of rectal bleeding. Figure 10.1 shows a suggested pattern of investigation. It should be noted that distinction can be made between the patient with any form of blood loss *not* accompanied by diarrhoea and those with bloody diarrhoea whether it be of long or short duration. In the latter situation, stool culture is the first priority in all such patients with, in addition, serological studies used selectively in those with a short history suggesting an acute infective aetiology.

Bloody diarrhoea of longer duration is most likely to be due to inflammatory bowel disease. Sigmoidoscopic appearances may suggest whether this is ulcerative colitis or Crohn's colitis, but final confirmation will rest on a histologist's report on biopsies taken. It should be noted that Crohn's colitis less commonly causes blood loss.

All other patients require investigation by means of rectal examination followed by proctosigmoidoscopy. Where a benign and treatable cause is found in a patient under the age of 45 years then it is reasonable not to investigate the bowel further, providing that after treatment there is no further blood loss.

In those over the age of 45 years this is not a safe course to pursue and full investigation is necessary even when a local cause for blood loss is demonstrated. Several studies of older patients with rectal bleeding and haemorrhoids have shown a significant yield of synchronous pathology higher up the bowel. A report from Israel showed that 45 of 194 patients with haemorrhoids had coexisting disease, including 12 cancers, 28 polyps, 4 inflammatory bowel disease, and 1 angiodysplasia. Another study from Hong Kong found 30 cancers in 337 patients aged over 40 years

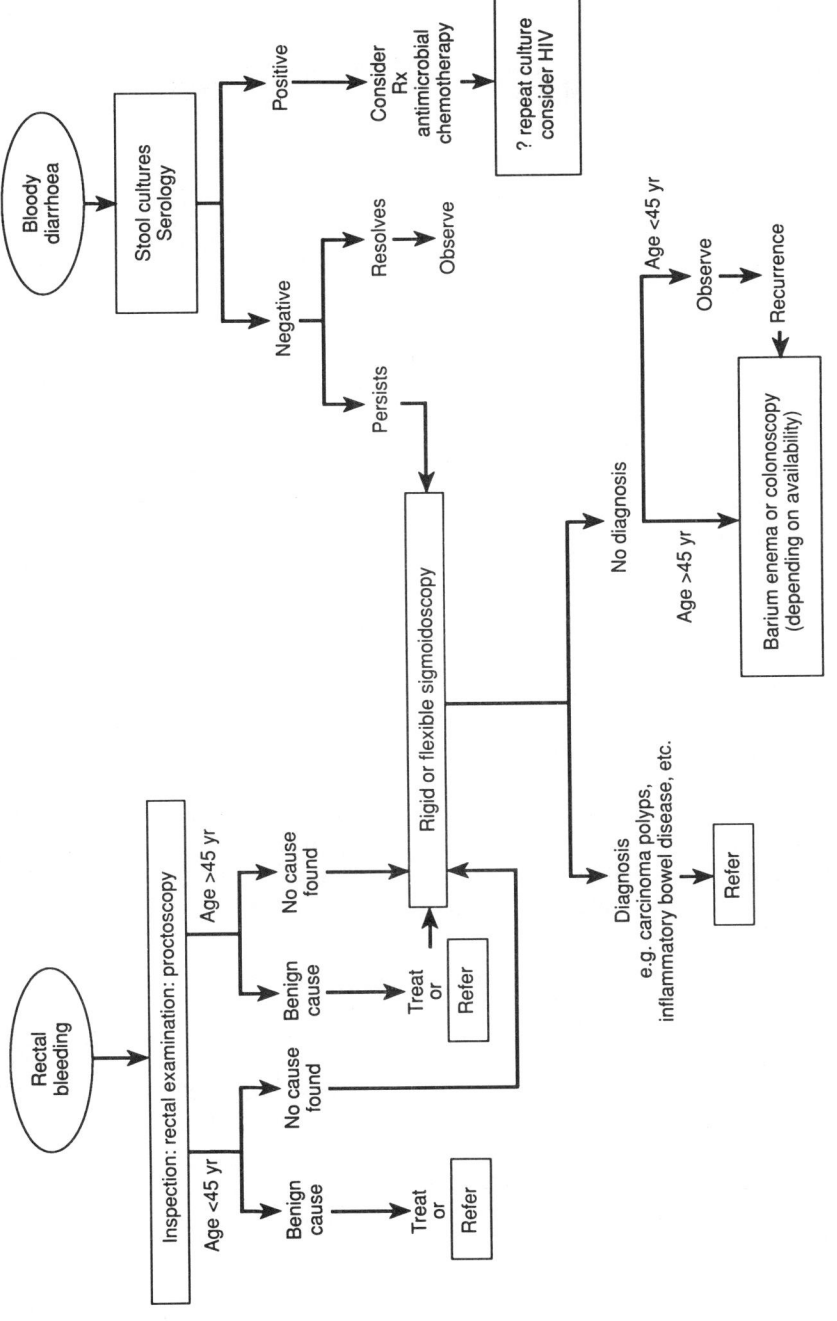

Fig. 10.1 The management of rectal bleeding.

investigated for rectal bleeding with an overall diagnostic yield of 29 per cent and concluded that patients with rectal bleeding should be screened for left-sided colon cancer irrespective of the clinical diagnosis.

The message here is quite clear—do not accept a diagnosis of haemorrhoids in a patient over the age of 45 years without investigating the colorectum.

THE MANAGEMENT OF CONDITIONS ASSOCIATED WITH RECTAL BLEEDING

Local anal disease

Perianal pruritis and excoriation (skin tags)

Constant itching and soreness of the anus causes the patient to scratch both by day and by night. It is important to exclude local infection, particularly with thrush and also infestation with thread worms. Eczematization of the perianal area may occur in susceptible individuals and psoriasis may affect the perianal area and and is often difficult to treat effectively. Any cause of discharge, vaginal or anal, requires correction. Anal leakage may arise because of impaired continence as a result of previous anal surgery or following episiotomy or childbirth trauma. Prolapsing haemorrhoids, anal fissures or fistulae will also cause anal wetness.

Treatment of perianal pruritis should first be directed to removal of any causes, coupled with scrupulous hygiene. This includes washing and drying of the area after defecation and the wearing of loose-fitting and absorbent underwear. Complete drying is essential and can best be achieved by use of a hair dryer held away from the anus. The local application of small quantities of hydrocortisone cream for a limited period usually breaks the cycle of itching and scratching. A strong psychological overlay may develop in some patients who relieve their life's frustrations on their long-suffering perianal region with dire consequences.

Thrombosed perianal vein (perianal haematoma or external pile)

If seen early this will present as a small tender perianal lump covered by skin. It can be incised radially if pain is severe but is more usually left alone. Frequent application of creams incorporating a local anaesthetic, such as Anugesic or Proctosedyl, ease the discomfort which usually last a few days. The patient should be warned that the lump may burst spontaneously, discharging blood clot.

Anal fissure

Superficial anal fissure of recent onset which is not associated with underlying disease may respond to conservative measures. These include the use of local anaesthesia in the form of suppositories or ointment (Anugesic/Proctosedyl) or the application of 2 per cent lignocaine gel via an applicator introduced into the anus. It is important to avoid the passage of hard constipated stools. This may be achieved by use of laxatives such as lactulose, senna, or a faecal softener, such as docusate sodium, with additional dietary fibre. If the patient does not obtain relief in a few days then surgical referral with a minimum of delay is appropriate.

Acute fissures which do not resolve with conservative measures, and all chronic and indurated fissures, will require surgical intervention. This may take the form of controlled anal dilatation under general anaesthesia or sphincterotomy with or without excision of the fisure.

Ano-rectal suppuration and fistulae

Ano-rectal suppuration may arise in a number of sites, the most common being a perianal abscess which collects just beneath the perianal skin. Similarly, pus may collect beneath the mucosa of the anal canal. Pus may also collect in the ischiorectal fat, spreading outwards from a fissure or a perianal abscess. From each of these sites pus may track either to the perianal skin surface or into the anal canal or rectum. Immediate surgical referral is necessary.

Haemorrhoids (piles)

First-degree haemorrhoids which cause acute symptoms usually respond to attention to diet with a view to correcting constipation and consequent straining; in particular an increase in roughage content and fluid intake with, in addition, the application of a simple emollient cream, such as Anusol. There are several similar preparations which contain in addition a local anaesthetic and hydrocortisone. These may be more comforting used in the short term, but it must be remembered that local anaesthetics can sensitize and then produce a considerable local reaction.

Injection therapy. More troublesome first-degree and second-degree haemorrhoids which are bleeding can be treated by injecting a sclerosant solution into the base of the haemorrhoid in order to promote fibrosis. This procedure, which may need to be repeated, will have no effect on prolapse, but does obliterate blood loss and promotes shrinkage of the anal cushions.

Rubber banding. The application of elastic rubber bands to second-degree and moderate sized third-degree haemorrhoids is a most effective way of treating them without recourse to surgery with general anaesthesia. Fortunately haemorrhoids arise from above the pectinate line and so do not have pain fibres. It is possible to apply several bands at a time via a suitable sized proctoscope. The base of the haemorrhoid is grasped with forceps and a very strong rubber band is applied so that its blood supply is obstructed, leading to infarction and eventual sloughing. This, in turn, leaves an area of ulceration which heals by scarring, causing mucosal fixation and a debulking of each anal cushion in turn.

Both injection therapy and elastic band ligation are suitable procedures to be carried out in general practice once experience has been gained. Injection therapy is considered to be an eligible procedure for minor surgery payment but illogically this is not yet so for banding haemorrhoids.

Surgical treatment.   Patients with large third-degree haemorrhoids and those in whom injection or elastic band ligation has not proved effective require referral for surgical assessment. The most usual procedure is admission for excision and low ligation under general anaesthesia.

INFLAMMATORY BOWEL DISEASE

An important cause of bleeding from the gastrointestinal tract is inflammation of the large bowel. Severe inflammation can lead to epithelial disruption and, ultimately, ulceration. Inflammatory diseases may be categorized into (1) *specific* inflammatory bowel disorders which consist of the colo-rectal infections in which we know the precise aetiological agent and (2) *non-specific* inflammatory bowel diseases, such as ulcerative colitis and Crohn's disease in which the aetiology remains obscure. Both types of inflammatory bowel disease are important world-wide, although their geographical distribution varies. Nevertheless, the increasing reports of infective colitis in the industrialized world and the increasing recognition of non-specific inflammatory bowel disease in the developing world make this a challenging area for clinicians.

Infective proctocolitis

This is the most common cause of colonic inflammation of the bowel in the developing world and is almost invariably the result of bacterial or parasitic infection (Tables 10.1 and 10.2). However, there are increasing reports of *Campylobacter* spp., *Salmonella* spp., and enterohaemorrhagic *E. coli* infections in the West. *E. histolytica*, the cause of amoebiasis, is endemic in many Western countries, including the UK, and travel abroad is unnecessary to acquire this infection, although primary infections in the UK are uncommon. Travellers to the developing world will be exposed to many of these enteropathogens, even schistosomiasis, which has been acquired by travellers who swim in Lake Victoria in East Africa. Another

Table 10.1 *Enteropathogens causing bloody diarrhoea*

Bacteria
  Shigella spp.
  Salmonella spp.
  Enteroinvasive *E. coli*
  Enterohaemorrhagic *E. coli*
  Campylobacter jejuni
  Yersinia enterocolitica
  C. difficle
  M. tuberculosis
  Aeromonas spp.
  Plesiomonas spp.

Protozoa
  Entamoeba histolytica
  Balantidium coli

Viruses
  Cytomegalovirus (in immunosuppressed patients)

Helminths
  Schistosoma spp.
  Trichuris trichiura (Whipworm)

Table 10.2 *Microbial agents causing proctitis and other inflammatory conditions of the ano-rectum*

Neisseria gonorrhoeae
Chlamydia trachomatis (LGV*)
Chlamydia trachomatis (non-LGV)
Treponema pallidum
Herpes simplex virus

* LGV, lymphogranuloma venereum.

major risk group is individuals with immunodeficiency, particularly those infected with HIV. Transmission of enteropathogens is generally via food or drink, but person-to-person spread is also important, including transmission as a result of some forms of sexual activity.

The clinical presentation may be either that of (1) proctitis or (2) a more extensive proctocolitis. Infective proctitis can be asymptomatic but will often present as a bloody rectal discharge. Associated symptoms include perineal discomfort and constipation. When the proctocolitis is more extensive, diarrhoea usually accompanies rectal bleeding and is commonly associated with quite severe lower abdominal cramping pain and fever. Unlike the acute small bowel enterotoxin-mediated infections, stool volumes in dysentery are usually relatively small. In cases of established *Shigella* colitis, the stools are bloody and mucoid and not watery. Infective colitis can be complicated by massive bleeding, toxic dilatation, and specific complications such as amoebic liver abscess, and in severe infection with *S. dysenteriae* type 1 infection, the haemolytic uraemic syndrome.

An aetiological agent should always be pursued in bloody diarrhoea. Proctosigmoidoscopy will confirm whether the inflammatory process is limited to the rectum or extends beyond and a biopsy may assist the diagnosis by detecting a specific enteropathogen such as *E. histolytica* trophozoites or the ova of *Schistosoma* spp. Proctosigmoidoscopy and rectal biopsy may be entirely normal, as infective colitis may be predominantly right-sided. Histologically it can be extremely difficult to distinguish infective colitis from non-specific inflammation. It is therefore essential to send at least three stool specimens for microscopic examination and culture. *E. histolytica* trophozoites are fragile and do not survive for long outside the human host. A fresh faecal specimen is therefore required. If antibiotic-related colitis due to *Clostridium difficile* is considered a possibility, faeces should also be sent for estimation of *C. difficile* toxin. Serology is surprisingly unhelpful in the diagnosis of intestinal infections, although at least 75 per cent of patients with active amoebic colitis will have a positive IgG antibody test. In acute schistosomal infection the specific enzyme-linked immunosorbent assay (ELISA) test will be positive is more than 95 per cent of infected individuals, but serology is of limited value in endemic areas as the test remains positive for many years even after eradication of the parasite.

The majority of intestinal dysenteric infections are self-limiting and other than restoration of water and electrolyte losses, specific therapy is generally not required. However, metronidazole should be given for amoebic colitis and antibiotics are required for *S. dysenteriae* infection (co-trimoxazole, nalidixic acid or ciprofloxacin). Other *Shigella* spp., *Salmonella* spp., and *Campylobacter* spp. infections usually resolve, but antibiotics given early in the illness may reduce the duration and severity. Antibiotics however, should be given if there is a systemic illness with high fever, prostration, and severe abdominal pain. Anti-diarrhoeal drugs should be avoided because of concerns that they precipitate toxic dilatation. However, the evidence supporting this concern is not well established.

Infective proctocolitis is potentially avoidable if appropriate measures are taken to limit exposure through the usual transmission routes. Antibiotic prophylaxis is not generally recommended, although it may be appropriate to consider ciprofloxacin or another 4-fluoroquinolone drug in individuals who are considered to be at high risk. Vaccines for many of the agents causing bacterial dysentery are under development, but as yet none are available for routine use.

Non-specific inflammatory bowel disease

Non-specific inflammatory bowel disease (Table 10.3), such as ulcerative colitis and Crohn's disease, can often resemble infective disorders, and thus it is always essential to exclude an entropathogen not only at first presentation but during subsequent relapses. In addition to the two major inflammatory bowel diseases there are some rarer conditions, such as collagenous colitis and microscopic colitis, which generally present with diarrhoea without bleeding. Behçet's disease can also include an ileocolitis but the endoscopic appearances and histology are not specific and diagnosis generally rests on the presence of other features of the syndrome, such as oral and genital ulceration, uveitis, and seronegative arthritis.

Ulcerative colitis and Crohn's disease are often distinguishable clinically, endoscopically, radiologically, and histologically, although in approximately 15 per cent of cases it is not possible to attribute the case to one or other disease classification and the term 'indeterminate colitis' is used. Clinical patterns of presentation are largely dependent on the extent of the disease. When disease is limited to the rectum (proctitis), bleeding is the predominant symptom, often associated with constipation. Anorectal involvement with Crohn's disease may be associated with particular perianal problems, such as anal skin tags, fistulae, fissures, perianal or ischiorectal abscesses, and excoriation of the perianal skin. Strictures may develop in the anorectum following chronic involvement. Perianal sepsis in Crohn's disease can be most debilitating and in advanced cases destruction of the anal sphincter can result in leakage or overt incontinence.

Table 10.3 *Non-specific inflammatory bowel diseases involving the colon and rectum*

Ulcerative colitis
Crohn's disease
Collagenous colitis
Microscopic colitis
Behçet's disease
Diversion colitis

With more extensive colonic involvement the symptom of diarrhoea becomes more predominant. In ulcerative colitis the disease is always in continuity, progressing proximally from rectum to caecum, whereas the distribution in Crohn's disease is highly variable; involvement of the right colon and caecum is most common.

Ulcerative colitis and Crohn's disease can present as a severe fulminant colitis with fever, abdominal pain and tenderness, and toxic dilitation of the colon. This occurs less commonly with Crohn's disease, although localized perforation with paracolic abscess and either internal or external fistulation are characteristic features. Both forms of non-specific chronic inflammatory bowel disease are associated with extra-intestinal manifestations, including skin problems (erythema nodosum, pyoderma gangrenosum), arthralgia, oral ulceration (particularly Crohn's disease), and inflammatory eye conditions (uveitis, episcleritis).

Diagnosis of chronic inflammatory bowel disease is based on a combination of clinical history, physical examination, radiology and/or endoscopy, and histology. Once an infective aetiology has been excluded, the severity and extent of the disease should be assessed. Diagnosis can often be made on sigmoidoscopy and biopsy alone. If the typical appearances of ulcerative colitis are present, namely loss of vascular pattern, contact bleeding or spontaneous bleeding, and if the upper limit of disease can be seen through the sigmoidoscope then no further investigation is required. In Crohn's disease the changes in the rectum and distal colon are likely to be discontinuous, with erythema, aphthoid ulcers or deeper linear ulcers abutting directly with normal appearing mucosa. A biopsy should be performed to confirm the endoscopic diagnosis. When diarrhoea is a predominant symptom and more extensive disease is suspected, it is usually helpful to assess the extent by colonoscopy or barium enema. In inflammatory bowel disease, colonoscopy is favoured because of the added advantage of being able to examine the terminal ileum and to take biopsies from ileum to rectum. However, an unprepared 'instant' barium enema can provide extremely useful information without the necessity for preparation of the colon and a return visit to the radiology department. In sick patients, neither investigation is recommended but useful information is often obtained from a plain abdominal radiograph. Colonic inflammation is usually indicated by the absence of faecal residue; the presence of colonic dilatation would raise alarms about the severity of the disease. In suspected Crohn's disease, an abnormal small bowel follow-through examination would clearly distinguish the disease from ulcerative colitis.

Treatment strategies for chronic inflammatory bowel disease depend on the extent and severity of the condition. In some instances treatment varies depending on whether the primary diagnosis is ulcerative colitis or Crohn's disease, although, in general, both diseases are treated with the same classes of drugs.

Proctitis

When disease is limited to the rectum or distal sigmoid colon, topical therapy with 5-aminosalicylic acid (5-ASA) or corticosteroid suppositories or enemas is appropriate. 5-ASA drugs are as effective as corticosteroids and can be used as first line therapy. For perianal and anorectal Crohn's disease, additional measures are used, including antibiotics such as metronidazole and corticosteroid creams for inflamed external lesions. Surgical drainage may be required for septic complications.

More extensive colitis

For mild or moderate disease, systemic therapy is usually advised, again using either an oral 5-ASA preparation (slow or delayed release mesalazine, olsalazine) or oral prednisolone, depending on severity. The 5-ASA drugs have an important contribution to make in maintenance of remission. There is no proven benefit of using corticosteroid drugs for maintenance therapy and these should therefore be used in short courses with gradual withdrawal over a period of 6–8 weeks. Some patients with Crohn's disease, however, do feel that a small dose of corticosteroid helps maintain remission, and thus in these instances the drug can be continued at a dose of, ideally, less than 10 mg/day.

For severe disease, hospitalization is required to enable administration of intravenous fluids, intravenous corticosteroids, and surveillance of the calibre of the colon. For severe disease which is unresponsive to standard therapy with corticosteroids, cyclosporin can be used, as this has recently been shown to benefit some patients with refractory ulcerative colitis. Other second line drugs, such as methotrexate, are also under evaluation.

Maintenance therapy with 5-ASA based drugs has been used for many decades and recent evidence suggests that this may also be of value in increasing the disease-free interval after surgery in Crohn's disease. Azathioprine is also of value in both ulcerative colitis and Crohn's disease as a steroid-sparing agent and for remission maintenance.

Failure to respond to medical therapy for severe acute colitis, particularly when associated with colonic dilatation or perforation, necessitates sub-total colectomy and ileostomy. In ulcerative colitis continuity can be restored at a later stage by construction of an ileoanal pouch anastomosis. This operation is not appropriate for patients with Crohn's diesease. Surgery may also be required for severe, intractable bleeding from the colon and for chronic ill-health related to persistently active disease despite full medical therapy. In children and adolescents, chronically active disease can produce growth retardation which can also be an indication for surgery. In long-standing extensive colitis the presence of a carcinoma or severe persistent dysplasia would be an indication for colectomy.

EQUIPMENT FOR USE IN GENERAL PRACTICE

Proctoscope

Proctoscopes are available in a bewildering range of patterns, widths, and lengths. For most purposes the Naunton-Morgan proctoscope is preferable (dimensions 64 mm × 22 mm). As an additional benefit it accommodates the Thomson 'one man bander' (see below). A Naunton-Morgan proctoscope costs £72.00 (1992 prices).

Rigid sigmoidoscope

There are two commonly used patterns of rigid sigmoidoscope. The Lloyd-Davies and the Welch Allyn. The latter is the better instrument, being extremely robust and giving a better illumination. It has the additional benefit of a hinged window which does not fall off in use, also the excellent light source can be used for other purposes. The same instrument can be purchased with disposable shafts, but the light source is not interchangeable with the re-usable model.

A re-usable (19 mm diameter) Welch Allyn sigmoidoscope with halogen fibre light costs £393.00. A similar instrument with disposable shafts costs £257.00. Disposable shafts cost £14.50 for a box of ten (1992 prices).

Biopsy forceps

Several patterns of biopsy forceps are available and it is important to establish that the forceps are the correct length for the sigmoidoscope being purchased. Commonly used patterns are those designed by Chevalier Jackson, Patterson, and Lloyd-Davies.

Biopsy forceps cost £155.00 (Lloyd-Davies) to £195.00 (Chevalier Jackson) (1992 prices), depending on length and pattern.

Flexible sigmoidoscope

The flexible instrument in common use is the fully immersible Olympus OSF-2 which is 600 mm in length. This instrument is marketed in the UK by Keymed Ltd; the cost is £8500 complete with light source, biopsy forceps, and cytology brush (1992 price). Keymed also offer a useful maintenance contract for this equipment.

Further information can be obtained from Keymed Ltd, Keymed House, Stock Road, Southend-on-Sea, Essex SS2 5QH (telephone 0702 616333).

Equipment for banding haemorrhoids

There are two patterns of banding equipment. There are those which require two operators, one to hold the proctoscope in position and one to pull the haemorrhoid through the ligator and then apply the elastic band. Alternatively, in the surgery situation this is not always possible, and the Thomson 'one man bander' may be preferable. This instrument fits snugly into the Naunton-Morgan proctoscope, so that the instrument can be held with one hand while the haemorrhoid is withdrawn through the bander ring with the other. It is useful to have two or three banders already loaded before beginning the procedure. Standard haemorrhoid ligators cost £39.00 each and Thomson 'one man banders' cost £60.00 each (1992 prices). Suitable forceps for grasping the haemorrhoids are either McGill's laryngoscopy forceps or Irwin Moore's nasal turbinate forceps which cost about £50.00, alternatively a St George's pattern grasping forceps costs £26.00. A more than adequate supply of elastic bands cost £9.85 for 100 bands (1992 prices).

All the equipment mentioned above, with the exception of the flexible endoscope, can be obtained from Seward Medical, 131 Great Suffolk Street, London SE1 1PP (telephone 071 357 6527).

FURTHER READING

Antagnostides, A. A., Hodgson, H. J. F. and Kirsher, J. B. (eds) (1991). *Inflammatory bowel disease*. Chapman and Hall, London.

Bat, L., Pines, A., Rabau, M. and Niv, Y. (1985). Colonoscopic findings in patients with hemorrhoids, rectal bleeding and normal rectoscopy *Israel Journal of Medical Sciences*, **21**, 139–41.

Cheung, P. S. Y., Wong, S. K. C., Boey, J. and Lai, C. K. (1988). Frank rectal bleeding: a prospective study of the causes in patients over the age of 40. *Postgraduate Medical Journal*, **64**, 364–8.

Cox, T. (1991). Flexible sigmoidoscopy in general practice. *Royal College of General Practitioners Members' Reference Book, 1991*, College of General Practitioners, London, p. 345.

Dent, O. F., Goulston, K. J., Zubrzycki, J. and Chapuis, P. H. (1986). Bowel symptoms in an apparently well population. *Diseases of Colon and Rectum*, **29**, 243–7.

Donald, I. P., Fitzgerald-Frazer, J. S. and Wilkinson, S. P. (1985). Sigmoidoscopy/proctoscopy service with open access to general practitioners. *British Medical Journal*, **290**, 759–61.

Farthing, M. J. G. (1991). Prevention and treatment of travellers' diarrhoea. *Alimentary Pharmacology and Therapeutics*, **5**, 15–30.

Farthing, M. J. G., Du Pont, H. L., Guandalini, S., Keusch, G. T. and Steffen, R. (1992). Treatment and prevention of travellers' diarrhoea. *Gastroenterology International* (In press).

Gazzard, B. G. (ed.) (1990). Gastroenterological aspects of AIDS. *Baillière's Clinical Gastroenterology*, Vol. 4 (2). Baillière Tindall, London.

Goulston, K. and Dent, O. (1987). Rectal bleeding: when and how to investigate. *Australian Family Physician*, **16**, (4), 379–82.

Hennigan, T. W., Franks, P. J., Hocken, D. B. and Allen-Mersh, T. G. (1990). Rectal examination in general practice *British Medical Journal*, **301**, 478–80.

Silman, A. J., Mitchell, P., Nicholls, R. J., Macrae, F. A., Leicester, R. T. and Bartram, C. I. (1983). Self reported dark red bleeding as a marker comparable with occult blood testing in screening for large bowel neoplasms. *British Journal of Surgery*, **70**, 721–4.

Springall, R. W. and Todd, I. P. (1988). General practitioner referral of patients with lower gastrointestinal symptoms. *Journal of the Royal Society of Medicine*, **81**, 87–8.

Tate, J. J. T. and Royle, G. T. (1988). Open access colonoscopy for suspected colonic neoplasia. *Gut*, **29**, 1322–5.

11 Colorectal cancer: early detection and screening

Jeremy Barnes

Colorectal cancer is a common complaint which affects both sexes and has a generally poor prognosis. Unfortunately, this disease only produces symptoms late in its course and the patient often delays seeking advice. Even when advice is sought there may be further delay in achieving an accurate diagnosis.

In 1990 16 560 people in the UK died of cancer of the colon or rectum. Colorectal cancer accounts for about 13 per cent of all cancers and is the most common form of cancer in non-smoking men and second only to breast cancer in women. Colorectal cancer is a disease of affluence and is the second most common cancer in the West.

A significant number of sufferers present acutely, often with obstructive symptoms, and require emergency surgery with its attendant risks. Of the remaining patients, only 50 per cent are found to be suitable for potentially curative surgery. Of those who do receive such treatment, less than 40 per cent will survive for five years. At present less than 10 per cent of patients present with an early (Dukes A) lesion—where the tumour is confined to the bowel wall. In this situation the prognosis is excellent and the five-year survival approaches 90 per cent.

There is an evident need to improve the prognosis for colorectal cancer. This may be done either by detecting symptomatic disease at an earlier, and thus more treatable, stage, or by effective prevention of the disease process itself. While the latter is the ideal solution it is as yet not fully achievable. Such measures as are available will be considered later.

THE EARLIER DETECTION OF SYMPTOMATIC DISEASE

There are no clear-cut diagnostic symptoms which single out patients as having a high probability of colorectal cancer. Patients subsequently demonstrated to have colorectal cancer have often presented to their general practitioner with non-specific gastrointestinal symptoms providing their doctor with considerable diagnostic difficulty. Perhaps the best discriminator for organic disease is the passage of some form of recognizable blood per rectum (see Chapter 10). Other symptoms, such as abdominal pain, sometimes relieved by defecation, alteration of bowel habit, and the passage of wind or mucus, are much less significant and are more commonly the result of irritable bowel syndrome (see Chapter 8). A need to pass bowel motions at night is a useful indicator of organic disease. Loss of weight and unexplained anaemia are non-specific but worrying features suggesting advanced disease.

Physical examination

Physical examination, and in particular examination of the abdomen, may be helpful to demonstrate a mass, and a digital rectal examination is mandatory in patients presenting with symptoms suggesting lower bowel disease. Fifteen per cent of tumours are within the reach of the examining finger. Yet a study from St Mark's Hospital showed how few rectal examinations had been carried out on the patients referred from general practice. It is a sobering fact that 10–20 per cent of patients with colorectal cancer have received treatment for haemorrhoids from their general practitioner in the two years preceding their diagnosis. The timescale for the development of cancer is such that a lesion was likely to have been present at that time.

Proctoscopy

Proctoscopy with an adequate light source will provide useful, although limited, information about the lower rectum and will demonstrate anal abnormalities and in particular the presence and severity of haemorrhoids.

INVESTIGATION

If the prognosis for patients with colorectal cancer is to be improved then general practitioners will have to lower their threshold of suspicion for cancer of the large bowel, so that in addition to a careful history and examination they will readily refer appropriate patients for further investigation. General practitioners are constantly being presented with non-specific gastrointestinal symptoms and have to make difficult decisions about who should be selected for investigation. It is worth emphasizing that colorectal cancer is a disease of later life and that the incidence of cancer doubles with each decade after the age of 40 years. Thus the age of the patient is an important determinant for referral.

Faecal occult blood tests in the symptomatic patient

There is a good case for a screening test for faecal occult blood, such as

Haemoccult, to be offered to all those patients with bowel-related symptoms where referral for further investigation is not otherwise certain. It should be emphasized that such a test is only a screening procedure and is not diagnostic of anything. It has a considerable false negative rate for cancer. The main value of such a test is that by its use some patients may be referred for investigation whose symptoms alone might not otherwise suggest referral.

Sigmoidoscopy

There is general agreement that investigation should begin with some form of inspection of the lower bowel prior to a double contrast barium enema. Unfortunately, there is a considerable variation in the availability of diagnostic facilities in different regions of the country. While some general practitioners may have direct access to departments of endoscopy which can offer either rigid or flexible sigmoidoscopy for their patients, in many other districts there is no such access and all patients have to be referred to a consultant at out-patients with the likelihood of extra delay in diagnosis. A consequence of a lack of direct access is that the general practitioner's threshold for referral may be raised and, because there is sometimes more ready access to contrast radiology, this may be used without prior sigmoidoscopy. Even a double contrast barium study of good quality is not a reliable method of diagnosing cancer of the rectum and sigmoid, which are the most common sites for colorectal tumours to present. The most obvious solution to this problem is for the profession to continue to press for open access to sigmoidoscopy.

There is, however, another valid approach, which is for practices to purchase and use their own instruments (see Chapter 2). This is more feasible in group practice, where a single partner can provide an in-house service to the practice as a whole, and of course the initial cost can be shared. By this means enough procedures will be carried out each year to maintain a certain level of expertise. Several general practitioners have appointments as hospital practitioners or clinical assistants in departments of endoscopy and are experienced in the use of flexible fibre-optic instruments. There are now a small number of practices in the UK that make use of these skills and provide a flexible sigmoidoscopy service for their patients.

As yet, there is no financial encouragement for practices to purchase and use sigmoidoscopes, but recent moves by the Department of Health suggest that this may change in the future. The use of a flexible sigmoidoscope has several advantages. It allows examination as far as the splenic flexure and thus identification of about 60 per cent of colorectal tumours. By contrast, a rigid instrument which really only examines the rectum can identify only 30 per cent of bowel tumours. Flexible sigmoidoscopy is much more acceptable to the patient than colonoscopy and patients do not normally require sedation or any form of aftercare.

Air contrast barium enema

Sigmoidoscopy should be followed by referral for air contrast barium enema. Again, access for this investigation is not universal and representations need to be made to redress this situation (see Chapter 2).

Colonoscopy

The place of colonoscopy in the early diagnosis of colorectal cancer is ill-defined. There is no doubt that this is the most accurate method of investigating the lower bowel and combines the benefits obtained by both sigmoidoscopy and contrast radiology with a greater diagnostic accuracy. It also provides the facility for taking tissue biopsies and removing small tumours by diathermy. Colonoscopy services are at present limited and are likely to remain so for some time to come. It is an expensive investigation which patients find unpleasant in spite of intravenous sedation. Colonoscopy is not without risk and is a procedure which requires an experienced operator with good facilities and trained nursing staff. Even in ideal circumstances this procedure has a definite morbidity and a very small mortality.

PREVENTION

Primary prevention

Primary prevention of colorectal cancer is, as yet, not possible. We recognize that this is a disease with a strong environmental aetiology and it is likely that dietary factors play a large part in its causation. Dietary fibre appears to exert a protective effect against the development of colonic cancer. This may be due to a reduction in bowel transit time or there may be other factors, such as the effects of the fermentation of dietary fibre and the consequent release of short-chain fatty acids such as butyrate. Studies of the relationship of diet to the development of colorectal cancer are difficult to interpret. Most studies show a positive correlation of mortality rates for colorectal cancer with a diet rich in meat and fat and a low content of fibre and vegetables. It is known that the disease is more prevalent amongst affluent areas of the world, such as North America and Western Europe, and less so in the peoples of South America and the rural parts of Africa. It is also known that individuals take on the colorectal cancer risk of their new country when emigrating from areas of low to areas of high incidence.

Secondary prevention

Secondary prevention entails the identification of malignant disease at an early enough stage to ensure a cure. This may be by early detection, as previously mentioned. In addition, it encompasses the identification and removal of premalignant lesions. The latter can be achieved either by case finding, that is by offering screening to patients attending their doctor for other reasons, or by some form of population screening. This may involve screening of whole populations or of identified groups which are known to be at greater risk than the general population.

In order to make decisions about which of these groups should receive screening it is necessary to consider the development of colorectal cancer as it is presently understood and look at the feasibility of secondary prevention.

Long-standing ulcerative colitis

Patients who have had ulcerative colitis for more than ten years are at increased risk of developing colorectal cancer and it is normal practice for them to be offered regular colonoscopic screening. In addition to visual inspection, biopsies are taken at different sites throughout the colon. These are screened for dysplasia; the presence of severe dysplasia is an indication for total colectomy.

Adenomatous polyps: the polyp-cancer sequence

The majority of colorectal cancers develop in pre-existing adenomatous polyps which are themselves extremely common. One in three of the UK population over the age of 50 years will have at least one colonic polyp. Both adenomatous polyps and carcinoma increase in frequency with age and polyps also increase in size with time. The evolution of colon cancer from adenomatous polyps is known as the polyp-cancer sequence. As polyps increase in size with time so they also have increased malignant potential. Polyps in excess of 2 cm diameter have a 50 per cent likelihood of malignancy. This progression is widely accepted, although the development of cancer in any particular polyp is by no means certain or inevitable and is at present poorly understood. There are at present only three factors known which may determine malignant change in an individual polyp. These are size, histological characteristics, and the degree of dysplasia.

Polypectomy

Fortunately colonic polyps stand out proud of the bowel mucosa and are easily seen via the endoscope. The majority can be readily and safely removed, either using biopsy forceps suitable for diathermy or by using a snare which is lassooed around the lesion and a diathermy current passed through the snare to cut off the lesion without blood loss. This can then be retrieved for histological section. Polyps vary considerably in size and the largest can prove difficult to remove, sometimes having to be removed piecemeal using snare diathermy.

Hyperplastic polyps

Otherwise known as metaplastic polyps, hyperplastic polyps consist of small foci of hyperplastic epithelial cells. They usually appear smaller and flatter than adenomatous polyps and are not thought to have malignant potential even though they are often seen in association with carcinoma of the rectum, presumably as a secondary phenomenon.

Colon cancer families

Although the development of colon cancer has a strong environmental aetiology, genetic factors have been demonstrated in family studies. There is a 2–4-fold increased risk of colorectal cancer in the first degree relatives of colorectal cancer sufferers, particularly where the patient is young. This risk also extends to relatives of patients with colonic adenomas. First degree relatives of patients with colorectal cancer or adenoma thus comprise a suitable higher risk group for screening.

A genetic basis for colorectal cancer

Recent developments in cytogenetics suggest that it may soon be possible to target screening at a selected population of susceptible individuals at high risk. This is already done in familial adenomatous polyposis (FAP) families; the numbers are very small and screening needs to be extended to cancer family syndrome and site specific cancer families, as discussed below.

It is now known that an abnormality of chromosome 5 is present in FAP. Where both copies of the relevant gene are lost in FAP individuals carcinoma inevitably develops. Of more importance for the population as a whole, it has been shown that in at least 20 per cent of cases of sporadic adenocarcinoma of the colorectum occurring in the general population there is absence of one of the alleles which are present in matched normal tissue. Thus, becoming recessive for this gene on chromosome 5 may be a critical first step in the development of a significant proportion of colorectal cancers. This discovery open the way for the future development of a test to identify susceptible individuals who can then be thoroughly screened.

Familial adenomatous polyposis (FAP)

This is a dominantly inherited condition occurring in 1 in 10 000 individuals in which those with the relevant gene develop vast numbers of polyps in their colon and rectum and to a lesser extent the rest of their gut. They have a 100 per cent chance of developing cancer often in their late teens or early twenties. It is essential that relatives of sufferers are screened by colonoscopy and biopsy soon after puberty. While this is an inherited disorder it should be remembered that up to 40 per cent of cases may be sporadic.

Cancer family syndrome and site-specific colon cancer

These are both hereditary non-polyposis family cancer syndromes and are difficult to recognize other than by their family pedigree, which demonstrates several first degree relatives with either colorectal cancer or with colorectal cancer and a variety of other adenocarcinomas. The risk of developing cancer in these families ranges from 1 in 17 for those having one affected relative to a 1 in 2 risk for those having three first degree relatives affected.

SCREENING

Screening of the colorectum could, in theory, utilize either a test for blood in the stool (faecal occult blood, FOB) as a first stage screen or involve visual inspection of the bowel with either a rigid or flexible endoscope. Population screening of low risk populations, whether on a case finding basis or by screening of a particular age group, involves such large numbers that any form of endoscopy as an initial procedure cannot be justified. By contrast, the screening of small groups at high risk, such as relatives of genetically determined cancer sufferers, can be carried out by initial total colonoscopy. Recent developments in cytogenetics make it likely that in the near future it may be possible to identify genetically susceptible individuals to refine still further those who require colonoscopy.

Faecal occult blood tests

Guiac tests (Haemoccult)

There are several FOB tests currently available in the UK and they vary both in quality and sensitivity as well as price. The most widely used test is Haemoccult, which is a dependable product with a standardized sensitivity. This test is used as a yardstick for other similar products and has also been used for most of the major screening studies world-wide. This test consists of a naturally occurring gum called guiac impregnated on to a filter paper. Hydrogen peroxide, when applied, acts as an oxidizing agent causing a blue coloration to occur in the presence of a catalyst. This reaction is catalysed by peroxidases and also by haematin released from haemolysed blood which has a pseudoperoxidase activity. A positive test depends on there being a sufficient quantity of haemolysed blood in the stool for it to become positive. The test is insensitive to blood from the proximal gastrointestinal tract, and since frank bleeding from the anus does not have time to haemolyse this does not give a positive test either. There is, however, a normal loss of blood from the bowel in healthy people and so the test has to be sufficiently insensitive to avoid giving false positive results. Items of normal diet, particularly fresh vegetables, may contain enough peroxidases to give false positive results, and larger amounts of blood of dietary origin may also give a false positive test. It might be thought that aspirin and NSAIDs provoke enough gastrointestinal blood loss to give a positive test leading to confusion and unnecessary investigation. However, in a study of nearly 11 000 people undergoing faecal occult blood screening. It was shown that occult bleeding cannot be attributed to upper gastrointestinal blood loss caused by NSAIDs, and that all such patients should undergo a thorough colorectal examination.

Large doses of vitamin C have a contrary effect, acting as a reducing agent and may provide a false negative result. Oral iron poses no problem. Some experts advise dietary restriction prior to testing for occult bleeding. While this may be sensible in the symptomatic patient it is probably counter-productive in the context of screening the asymptomatic population because of its effect on compliance.

Immunological tests (Haemselect)

These tests are a more recent innovation and are still being assessed for use in Europe. They depend for their action on the use of mono-specific antisera to human haemoglobin and so are not affected by items of diet. As presently formulated these tests are more sensitive than Haemoccult, but increasing sensitivity has also reduced their specificity. This, in turn, has increased the number of false positive tests and the number of asymptomatic patients subjected to unnecessary investigation. At present such tests are more expensive and also more difficult to process, requiring technical expertise in order to achieve reliable results.

The use of FOB tests

Increased faecal blood loss is known to occur in most patients with colorectal neoplasia. The sensitivity of screening using Haemoccult to detect cancer varies with the site of the tumour, being of greater accuracy in detecting proximal colonic tumours. Sensitivity for adenomas is similarly affected and only the larger adenomas are likely to cause sufficient blood loss to give a positive test.

FOB tests may be used in the symptomatic or asymptomatic patient. As previously mentioned, a test may be used in patients with non-specific bowel symptoms who might not otherwise merit investigation and by this means neoplasia or inflammatory bowel disease may be diagnosed earlier. It must be emphasized, however, to both doctor and patient that a negative test is no guarantee of normality.

Screening of asymptomatic patients has to be targeted at a specific sub-population, usually defined by age criteria, to obtain the highest yield of disease for the outlay involved, in terms of patient commitment, medical input, and cost. Stool sampling is not popular with patients, who even today are embarassed by discussion of their bowel function and dislike contact with their faeces, so that good compliance is always a problem with such projects. It has been shown that the best uptake of FOB screening is achieved when the general practitioner personally offers the test opportunistically at the end of a consultation on another matter.

Several controlled studies of FOB screening using Haemoccult have been reported both from the USA and Europe. These studies have achieved compliance rates of 53–67 per cent and produced positive rates in asymptomatic individuals varying between 1.1 and 2.3 per cent. These results produced positive predictive values for cancer of 11–17 per cent and for adenoma of 36–41 per cent. These results are encouraging, but there is also a false negative rate to consider. In a study based in Nottingham involving 107 349 patients, 20 out of 98 cancers went undetected by the faecal occult blood test, a sensitivity of 77 per cent. This compares favourably with other series world-wide. An encouraging feature of this study is that 52 per cent of the cancers detected by screening were localized to the bowel wall (Dukes A) and thus had an excellent prognosis compared with the control group, where only 11 per cent of cancers were classified as Dukes A.

Screening in general practice

Opportunistic screening of the older age groups—for example, those over 50 years of age in the practice setting is feasible, particularly if the practice is able to carry out some of the necessary investigation of patients with positive tests in-house. It is necessary to negotiate a supply of Haemoccult from the District department of chemical pathology and to ensure its reliable processing either by the practice nursing staff or by delivery to the chemical pathologist. It is important to take a full history, particularly a family history of bowel diseases, from those with a positive test and then to

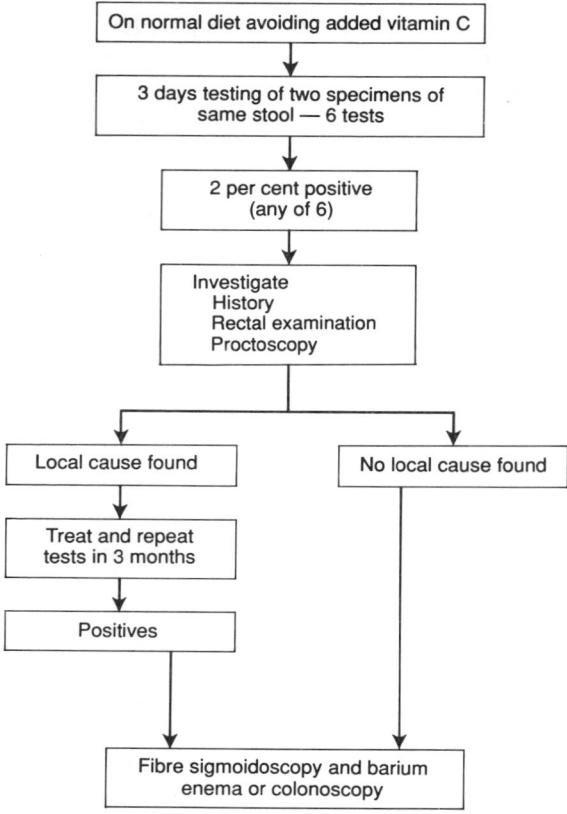

Fig. 11.1 Screening for colorectal cancer in the asymptomatic population.

carry out an examination including a digital rectal examination and proctoscopy. If a local cause for blood loss is found then it is wise to treat the cause and then repeat the test, since it is possible that the patient also has disease higher up the bowel to account for the positive test.

While colonoscopy is the investigation of choice it is unlikely to be readily available and in most districts a sigmoidoscopy—either rigid or flexible—followed by a barium enema is the norm (Fig. 11.1).

Such a process will produce a yield of about 2 per cent of patients with positive FOB tests, of whom about two thirds will be found to have either cancer or adenoma. Rescreening every two years will produce a much smaller yield. Because of the low sensitivity of the test, interval neoplasia will occur and it is essential that both patient and doctor are not lulled into ignoring bowel symptoms on the basis of a previous negative FOB test.

Table 11.1 *Screening for colorectal cancer in general practice*

A typical four doctor group practice, list size 8000, 25 per cent of patients are over 50 years old

Offer screening every two years to 1000 potential screenees each year

Initially a low uptake—lower by postal offer
   —higher by personal offer from general practitioner face to face

Haemoccult probably available from chemical pathology department, either for processing at department or at surgery

Maximum uptake will generate 20 positive tests for investigation in one year

---

Table 11.1 shows the logistics of such an undertaking in a typical group practice.

The value of FOB screening

Screening for colorectal cancer in common with all other screening strategies requires careful evaluation before implementation. Population screening using any form of endoscopy as a primary tool is not practical and the only possible method available at present is the use of faecal occult blood testing. As already mentioned the sensitivity and specificity of the tests in current use leave much to be desired and patient uptake is only about 60 per cent. Additional valuable information will be gained from the randomized controlled trials which are presently in progress. The results to date suggest that in contrast to symptomatic patients, cancers found in screened populations show a higher proportion of localized tumours (Dukes A) and are thus detected at an earlier stage in the progress of the disease. Unfortunately, it is not possible to simply assume that detection at an earlier stage proves the value of screening. Lead time and other biases may influence conclusions as to the apparent value of screening. At least the lesions are more amenable to treatment and a higher proportion of lesions can be dealt with endoscopically.

It is not yet possible to show whether screening improves either the duration or the quality of life. It is hoped that this information will become available from the Nottingham study in 1995. No national decision on the introduction of FOB population screening will be made before these results are available.

It is relevant to observe that doubt has been cast on the value of the existing national screening programmes for the detection of breast cancer and cervical cancer which were not so carefully evaluated before their

Table 11.2 *Incidence figures and death rates for cancer of the breast, cervix, and colorectum*

Carcinoma	Males	Females	Total
Incidence figures for 1985 in England and Wales			
Breast	177	22 064	22 241
Cervix	—	3970	3970
Colorectum	11 778	12 070	23 848
Death rates for 1990 in England and Wales			
Breast	107	13 634	13 741
Cervix	—	1781	1781
Colorectum	8189	8371	16 560

introduction. They may have been introduced in part for political expedience.

Table 11.2 compares the incidence and death rates for cancer of the breast, cervix, and colorectum in England and Wales. It is difficult to state the precise costs of the existing screening programmes, but it is estimated that the national cervical screening programme costs at least £30 million annually and at its inception it was expected that each year breast screening by mammography would cost £50 million, with a similar cost for the consequences of screening. No estimate has yet been made of the cost of a national colorectal cancer screening programme. Clearly, the initial screen using a faecal occult blood test, such as Haemoccult, would be of modest cost. However, the consequence of testing is that about 2 per cent of the population would require investigation and there will need to be a considerable expansion of endoscopic and radiological services to meet this need. Such an expansion would involve considerable investment in both medical manpower, facilities, and finance. In 1989 Hardcastle, working with an economist, estimated that the cost of screening the 75 000 people at risk of developing colorectal cancer in an average health district was approximately £250 000. This works out at a little over £2000 per cancer detected, which compares favourably with costs similarly calculated, of £3000 for each breast cancer detected by mammography and almost £3500 for each cervical cancer detected in the conventional cervical screening programme.

Polyp follow-up guide-lines

Screening studies, as described above, will identify large numbers of people with one or more polyps in their colon or rectum. In addition, there will be symptomatic patients whose investigation has revealed the presence of polyps. We know that polyps increase in size with time and that increasing size also increases the likelihood of malignant change. In addition, the histological characteristics of the adenoma and the degree of dysplasia present are also determinants of the likelihood of malignant transformation. Unfortunately, these parameters are fallible and as yet there is no clear picture as to who should be regularly reviewed and how often. The presence of polyps is no guarantee of the future development of malignant disease.

The King's Fund has recently considered the need for colonoscopic surveillance in these patients. They recommend that in symptomatic patients with a polyp the whole bowel is examined and polyps greater than 5 mm diameter are removed. They also advise against regular colonoscopy of patients with a single small tubular rectal adenoma or those aged over 75 years. They do, however, recommend that those with a large adenoma or any type of multiple adenoma should undergo colonoscopy every 3–5 years. The implications of these recommendations are formidable bearing in mind the present limited availability of colonoscopy.

In conclusion, it is likely that evidence will soon be available to demonstrate the value of screening for colorectal cancer in reducing both morbidity and mortality for a disease which otherwise has a high mortality and which has a high prevalence in the community. If such screening is introduced nationally it is likely that a large part of the burden will fall on general practitioners. It is essential that the full implication of this is understood and that adequate facilities and remuneration are arranged well in advance.

FURTHER READING

Ascari, A., Ponz de Leon, M., Antonioli, A., Bernardelli, D., Amorotti, C., Merighi, A. *et al.* (1986). Colorectal cancer among first-degree relatives of patients with cancer or polyps of the large bowel. *Italian Journal of Gastroenterology*, **18**, 52.

Gyde, S. (1990). Screening for colorectal cancer in ulcerative colitis: dubious benefits and high costs. *Gut*, **31**, 1089–92.

Hardcastle, J. D., Thomas, W. M., Chamberlain, J., Sheffield, J., Pye, G., James, P. D. *et al.* (1989). Randomised controlled trial of faecal occult blood screening for colorectal cancer: results for first 107 349 subjects. *Lancet*, **1**, 1160–4.

Hobbs, F. D. R., Cherry, R. C., Fielding, J. W. L., Pike, L. and Holder, R. (1992). Acceptability of opportunistic screening for occult gastrointestinal blood loss. *British Medical Journal*, **304**, 483–6.

Lovett, E. (1976). Family studies in cancer of the colon and rectum. *British Journal of Surgery*, **63**, 13–18.

MacPherson, A. J. S., Bjarnason, J. and Forgacs, I. C. (1992). Discovery of the gene for familial adonomatous polyposis. *British Medical Journal*, **304**, 858–9.

Mant, D., Fuller, A., Northover, J., Astrop, P., Chivers, A., Crockett, A. *et al.* (1992). Patient compliance with colorectal cancer screening in general practice. *British Journal of General Practice*, **42**, 18–20.

Morson, B. C. (1976). Genesis of colorectal cancer. *Clinical Gastroenterology*, **5**, 505–25.

Murday, V. (1990). The family cancer clinic. In *Screening for colorectal cancer*. Proceedings of an International Meeting organized by the UK Coordinating Committee on Cancer Research (ed. J. D. Hardcastle), Normed Verlag, Bad Hamburg, Hamburg.

Pollock, A. M. and Quirke, P. (1991). Adenoma screening and colorectal cancer. *British Medical Journal*, **303**, 3–4.

Pye, G., Ballantyne, K. C., Armitage, N. C. and Hardcastle, J. D. (1987). Influence of non-steroidal anti-inflammatory drugs on the outcome of faecal occult blood tests in screening for colorectal cancer. *British Medical Journal*, **294**, 1510–11.

Solomon, E., Voss, R., Hall, V., Bodmer, W.F., Jass, J. R., Jeffreys, A. J. *et al.* (1987). Chromosome 5 allele loss in human colorectal carcinomas. *Nature*, **328**, 617–19.

Springall, R. W. and Todd, I. P. (1988). General practitioner referral of patients with lower gastrointestinal symptoms. *Journal of the Royal Society of Medicine*, **81**, 87–8.

Stemmermann, G. N., Nomura, A. M. Y. and Heilbrun, L. K. (1984). Dietary fat and the risk of colorectal cancer. *Cancer Research*, **44**, 4633–7.

12 The care of gastrointestinal cancer

Wendy Makin

Gastrointestinal malignancy accounts for more than 39 000 cancer deaths in England and Wales each year, out of a total of 140 000. During the past 30 years there has been little change in the number of people presenting and dying with colorectal cancer; the number with gastric cancer has fallen, only to be matched by an increase in pancreatic neoplasms. The sad fact remains that despite efforts to develop new and existing curative treatments, the majority of people with these cancers will still die from their disease. In practical terms for the general practitioner, the management of patients with advanced disease is a greater problem than dealing with those with early malignancy. With this in mind, this chapter gives a synopsis, not only of the current approaches aimed at cure, but also of palliative measures and the indications for their use.

OESOPHAGEAL CANCER

Oesophageal malignancies accounted for 4334 cancer registrations in England and Wales in 1984 and cause around 4000 deaths annually; the overall five-year survival for all cases is only 5 per cent.

Oesophageal cancer is linked to smoking and alcohol intake and there is an established association with iron deficiency anaemia and achalasia. By far the most common tumours are squamous carcinomas; adenocarcinomas which arise in the lower third of the oesophagus account for only 6 per cent. Very rare malignacies include melanoma, sarcomas, and small cell carcinomas similar to those in the bronchial tree.

Spread is by longitudinal submucosal infiltration with early lymphatic invasion to the mediastinal, supraclavicular, and upper abdominal nodes. At a later stage, direct invasion of adjacent structures, for example left main bronchus or pericardium occurs. Bone, lung, and liver are the distant sites most frequently involved by haematogenous spread. Occasionally, squamous carcinomas are responsible for paraneoplastic phenomena, such as clubbing, hypercalcaemia or myoneuropathies.

The majority of patients complain of progressive difficulty in swallowing, first solids then liquids, and often they can localize the level of obstruction. There may be discomfort due to oesophagitis, but persistent chest pain may indicate tumour infiltration beyond the oesophagus. Regurgitation of food is common and aspiration of liquids may lead to pneumonia. By the time of diagnosis, weight loss is marked and there may be anaemia due to occult blood loss or occasionally brisk haematemesis.

The poor prognosis for most cases of oesophageal cancer is associated with a late stage of disease at diagnosis: dysphagia may not be significant until more than half the circumference of the oesophagus is involved. There is evidence of distant metastatic spread in up to one third of patients at diagnosis.

Barium studies together with endoscopic assessment and biopsy are essential investigations; CT scans may be useful to exclude paraoesophageal extension or lymphadenopathy when radical treatment is contemplated. Macroscopic tumours greater than 5 cm in length are usually associated with positive nodes and as such are unlikely to be curable.

The presence of palpable neck nodes, hoarseness due to a recurrent laryngeal nerve palsy, or an epigastric mass, all indicate advanced malignancy. However, severe cachexia in the absence of other signs does not confer a hopeless prognosis, but reflects the severity and duration of difficulties in swallowing. These patients still warrant full assessment.

MANAGEMENT OF EARLY OESOPHAGEAL CANCER

Due to late presentation and diagnosis, only about half the patients are suitable for radical surgery. The tumour is resected with a wide margin and continuity of the gastrointestinal tract restored. The approach and site of the anastamosis will depend upon the level of the tumour, but operative mortality is around 20 per cent, lower third resections usually carrying less risk of complications. The results in terms of cure are disappointing, with most patients surviving for less than one year after surgery. The outlook is best for patients with completely resected tumours and uninvolved lymph nodes, 20–30 per cent of whom will survive for five years.

High-dose radical radiotherapy can cure carefully selected patients where the carcinoma appears to be confined to the oesophagus and extends no more than 5–6 cm. It is particularly useful for treatment of the mid to upper oesophagus and provides an alternative to pharyngolaryngectomy for post-cricoid carcinoma, but surgery is usually preferable for lower third lesions. Postoperative radiotherapy is occasionally indicated for microscopically residual disease at the resection line, but there is no survival benefit if it is given to cases with involved nodes. No large trials have yet been completed which compare the results of radiation treatment with surgery. Radical radiotherapy achieves an overall five-year survival rate of 9 per cent, rising to 20 per cent for post-cricoid cancer, and these figures include many cases who would be considered unfit for an operation.

All patients who are to undergo radical treatment of either type require prior correction of dehydration, anaemia, and nutritional deficiencies. This may entail insertion of a central line for preoperative parenteral feeding, or the implementation of nasogastric feeds before and during irradiation. Although radiotherapy does not carry the high treatment-related mortality associated with surgery, all patients develop brisk radiation oesophagitis during treatment which often worsens the dysphagia and persists for some weeks.

Chemotherapy alone is not a curative treatment in oesophageal cancer, although several drugs, including methotrexate and cisplatin, produce response rates of over 40 per cent. Combined modality approaches, for example giving such drugs before surgery or radiation, may improve results, but this is still under investigation in clinical trials.

Patients who relapse after treatment will usually do so within the first two years. Further dysphagia does not inevitably imply recurrence: strictures occur in more than 20 per cent of cases following surgery and in up to 40 per cent after radiotherapy, so endoscopy is required to establish the cause. Repeated dilatations may be necessary for benign strictures. Post-thoracotomy pain may persist for months or years; sometimes application of a transcutaneous nerve stimulator (TENS) to the chest wall is effective. Sadly, many patients will relapse, either with local recurrence in the thorax or at distant sites. The development of a new chest pain or hoarseness together with dysphagia should be regarded with concern. Problems due to metastatic spread include bone pain, shortness of breath from pulmonary deposits or effusion, or anorexia and discomfort due to liver disease. Sometimes supraclavicular nodes appear in the asymptomatic patient.

MANAGEMENT OF ADVANCED OESOPHAGEAL CANCER

The majority of patients will present with incurable cancer because of either extensive primary disease or metastatic spread, and most of these will survive only 4–6 months. Any treatment of the oesophageal tumour can only be palliative and should be directed towards controlling symptoms without significant prolongation of life expectancy. Where dysphagia is the main problem, major surgery is clearly avoided in favour of simpler procedures which enable the patient to return home as soon as possible. When laparotomy has been undertaken in the hope of a curative operation, there is opportunity to perform a by-pass procedure which relieves dysphagia, but even this carries a high mortality risk. A more commonly used alternative is insertion of a Celestin tube which is pulled down through the narrowed oesophagus via a gastrotomy and has an expanded upper end to prevent displacement. Oesophageal intubation may be achieved at endoscopy using a guide-wire; this avoids laparotomy in patients with far advanced disease and is preferable to endoscopic dilatation alone, which may relieve dysphagia for only two weeks or less. Dilatation followed by intubation gives rapid relief and also blocks off fistulae, but is unsuitable for upper thoracic and cervical tumours. All intubation techniques are associated with a risk of perforation and a mortality rate of around 10–15 per cent, but when successful afford good palliation. Patients with tubes in place should be advised to maintain a soft diet, taking plenty of fluid with meals. Effervescent drinks are helpful in keeping the tube patent and hyoscine hydrobromide, 0.3 mg sublingually every 3–4 hours, reduces problems with saliva.

Repeated laser vaporization of tumour can improve luminal patency and relieves dysphagia in 70 per cent but also carries a potential hazard of perforation. Palliative radiotherapy may be given to patients with dysphagia, bleeding or pain due to invasion of paraoesophageal tissues, but is contraindicated if tumour is invading bronchus where there is a risk of fistula formation. Furthermore, radiotherapy is an important means of palliating metastatic disease, particularly bone deposits.

In addition to the familiar external beam techniques, intraluminal radiotherapy may be used in oesophageal cancer. This requires temporary intubation with a narrow applicator, which is passed through the malignant stricture. The applicator may then be loaded with miniaturized radioactive sources which deliver a high dose in the vicinity of the tumour. Treatment can be given in a single session lasting 20–30 minutes. Radiotherapy improves dysphagia in more than 50 per cent of patients; although there is transient oesophagitis, they are unlikely to survive long enough to develop strictures.

GASTRIC CANCER

There are more than 11 000 registrations of gastric cancer annually in England and Wales, with the number of deaths approaching 10 000. The overall five-year survival for this malignancy is 5–10 per cent.

More than 90 per cent of gastric cancers are adenocarcinomas; the remainder of rare tumours include leiomyosarcomas, plasmacytomas, and lymphomas. While there is an established association with achlorohydria and previous gastric surgery, dietary carcinogens are thought to be important in the aetiology, and presumably explain variation in geographical incidence. Fortunately the incidence of this cancer is falling in the West.

Gastric cancer invades the adjacent pancreas, spleen, and colon, and may extend into the lower oesophagus. In the UK, most cases have lymph node involvement at the time of surgery. Intraperitoneal spread is not uncommon, causing ascites, ovarian tumours, and masses in the pouch of Douglas. The majority of patients die from local disease rather than distant spread although liver metastases develop in 30 per cent, bone and lung deposits being less common.

The first symptoms may be anorexia or early satiety with weight loss. Nausea and vomiting or dysphagia may develop, while in some the presentation is through blood loss, either as iron deficiency anaemia or haematemesis. While only a small proportion of patients with dyspeptic symptoms will have gastric cancer, investigation of persistent indigestion, especially in people over 50 years of age, may reveal underlying malignancy. In Japan, where there is a particularly high incidence of gastric cancer, early investigation of rather non-specific symptoms has increased the proportion of early cases at diagnosis. Here patients often have a barium meal followed by endoscopy and biopsy and are found to have advanced malignancy: in one British series, only 27 per cent were operable at presentation.

MANAGEMENT OF EARLY GASTRIC CANCER

The surgeon hopes to achieve cure by complete resection of the tumour with its draining lymph nodes. This usually entails *en bloc* removal of the stomach, omentum, spleen, and part of the pancreas, plus lymphadonectomy. Sometimes a partial gastrectomy will be performed where the cancer is localized to the cardia. Perioperative mortality can be up to 30 per cent with radical surgery, which is offset by the chance of cure where there is early disease: this is more than 60 per cent if tumour is confined to the mucosa, dropping to less than 25 per cent when the serosa has been breached. Sadly the overall figure for all operable patients is around 15 per cent survival at five years. Attempts to improve these dismal results include more extensive lymph node dissection and the use of adjuvant chemotherapy. So far, trials of combined treatment have failed to show survival benefit. Further studies into the value of post-operative radiotherapy are in progress.

Patients with gastric lymphoma tend to have a better prognosis. These tumours occur in younger adults than most gastric cancer, and are often difficult to distinguish from carcinoma on endoscopic appearance alone. They may present with an acute bleed or perforation. Many gastric lymphomas are histologically high grade and cure is possible by combining resection with adjuvant chemotherapy; the five-year survival is more than 50 per cent.

More than half of all patients who have undergone radical surgery for adenocarcinoma will develop recurrence at the primary site; this may be associated with epigastric discomfort and a mass, sometimes with severe pain radiating to the back. Hepatomegaly and ascites are common features of advancing disease which is associated with marked cachexia.

MANAGEMENT OF ADVANCED GASTRIC CANCER

Palliative surgery has a useful role in resection of bleeding tumours or relief of obstruction, for example, a gastroenterostomy may be performed to by-pass an obstructing antral tumour. Radiotherapy has been infrequently used for inoperable gastric carcinomas; its use is limited by the poor tolerance of the upper abdomen to radiation. It is arguable whether radiotherapy has any effect on life expectancy, which is around six months; it is also associated with acute side-effects, particularly nausea and vomiting. Radiotherapy may be appropriate for a few patients with pain from recurrent tumour and whose general condition remains good, but it has no role in the treatment of widespread intra-peritoneal disease.

Several cytotoxic agents, including adriamycin, 5-fluorouracil, cisplatin, and mitomycin, produce short-term responses in gastric cancer. This is increased if a combination of agents is used, but any prolongation of survival in patients with inoperable disease must be carefully balanced against toxicity, visits to hospital and consideration of the overall quality of life of each individual.

Distension and discomfort due to malignant ascites may be a problem for these patients. Severe distension or discomfort requires paracentesis and this should be combined with diuretics: frusemide 40–80 mg daily with spironolactone 100–200 mg. Intra-peritoneal instillation of a cytotoxic drug, such as bleomycin, may reduce the need for further drainage without the systemic side effects of chemotherapy. Patients whose main problem is ascites and who are generally quite well could benefit from the insertion of a peritoneovenous shunt which permits circulation of ascitic fluid without the requirement for repeated paracentesis.

CANCER OF THE PANCREAS

Cancer of the pancreas accounts for around 6000 new registrations each year in England and Wales, and a similar number of deaths: barely 1 per cent of patients will survive for five years.

The pancreas is the site of a number of uncommon endocrine tumours which may arise as part of multiple endocrine neoplasia (MEN) syndromes and have familial associations. Most tumours however are adenocarcinomas, which are more common in smokers and in patients with diabetes of recent onset. Chronic pancreatitis is not a cause of malignancy, but may impede the diagnosis. A total of 60 per cent of tumours arise in the head of the pancreas, 20 per cent in the tail, and the rest in the ampullary region. There is local invasion of stomach, spleen, adrenal glands, and colon, and spread to the liver via the portal vein. Lymphatic invasion occurs at an early stage; by the time of surgery, 80 per cent have involvement of the regional nodes.

The early symptoms of pancreatic cancer are insidious: weight loss, upper abdominal discomfort, and complaints of feeling bloated. Between 50 and 80 per cent of patients have pain when they first seek advice. The pain is characteristically epigastric and often radiates through to the back; a few have backache alone. Severe pain radiating to the back implies inoperable disease and the poor prognosis for this malignancy is attributable to the regional or distant spread present in 85 per cent of cases at diagnosis. Obstructive jaundice develops in cancer arising in the head of the organ, but is preceded by pain in two thirds of patients. Other clinical problems encountered include obstruction of the duodenum and, occasionally, pancreatitis due to blockage of the papilla; diarrhoea can arise if there is obstruction to release of pancreatic enzymes. In up to 10 per cent, there is an associated migratory thrombophlebitis.

The diagnosis is reached with the aid of ultrasound scans or computerized tomography (CT), together with histological proof from fine needle aspiration or by cytology obtained at endoscopic retrograde pancreatography (ERCP).

TREATMENT OF EARLY PANCREATIC CANCER

Surgical resection offers the only, although slim, chance of cure but with considerable morbidity and risk of death from the procedure. The best results are achieved in patients with small (2 cm) tumours in the pancreatic head: up to 37 per cent five-year survival has been reached in these more fortunate, but proportionately few, patients. Those cancers arising in the tail are rarely resectable, and in most series only about 10 per cent of all patients are operable at laparotomy.

Whipples opeation is the established curative procedure: a radical pancreatoduodenectomy, leaving a pancreatic remnant which drains into a loop of jejunum. This is associated with a perioperative mortality of 20 per cent and even if resection is achieved, less than 20 per cent of patients are alive a year later. The overall cure rate achieved is 5–10 per cent, but most fail due to local recurrence. More extensive regional surgery, entailing a total pancreatectomy with dissection of the para-aortic nodes may improve the success rate; although the patient is thereafter inevitably insulin dependent, this does avoid anastamotic complications. In many patients postoperative steatorrhoea requires enzyme supplements combined with an H_2-receptor antagonist.

The site of the pancreas presents technical difficulties when attempting to deliver an effective dose of radiotherapy without exceeding the tolerance of surrounding structures. Radiation treatment may be used for inoperable cases but it remains secondary to surgery for early pancreatic cancer. Combined modality approaches incorporating either radiotherapy (sometimes delivered intraoperatively) or chemotherapy may improve local control. At present this should be confined to clinical trials.

The rare endocrine tumours include insulin-, glucagon-, and gastrin-secreting neoplasms which show a spectrum of benign to malignant behaviour. Surgery is the only curative treatment for early stage tumours, and at least reduces the bulk of peptide-producing tissue in other cases. Partial gastrectomy is sometimes performed in gastrinomas, where there is excessive tumour-induced acid secretion, if the site of the primary tumour cannot be found.

Hepatic metastases can be major source of peptide production and embolization of the hepatic artery, thus depleting the vascular supply to the tumour deposits, can effectively reduce symptoms. Chemotherapy, using agents such as 5-fluorouracil, adriamycin or streptozotocin, produces variable responses in different tumours, but is sometimes used in the palliation of symptomatic disease. The somatostatin analogue, octreotide, can also reduce peptide secretion.

MANAGEMENT OF ADVANCED PANCREATIC CANCER

When advanced disease is discovered at laparotomy, simpler procedures may be performed which will alleviate symptoms while carrying a lesser operative mortality. Most patients in this situation will survive only eight months from operation whichever surgical procedure is performed. The palliation of obstruction may be achieved through gastrojejunostomy and cholecysto-jejunostomy, while a coeliac block may be performed at laparotomy in cases where pain has been a presenting symptom.

Patients presenting with advanced disease in a state of poor health are not candidates for surgery. Radiotherapy can be used to palliate pain from inoperable tumour; it has been combined with chemotherapy in this situation. There is evidence to suggest that this may extend short-term survival, but has little impact upon overall survival. Radiotherapy is not helpful in alleviation of obstruction, whether intestinal or biliary. Jaundice may be effectively relieved by stenting of the ducts endoscopically or using a percutaneous, transhepatic method. When upper abdominal pain is a major problem, blockade of the coeliac plexus with injection of alcohol under radiological screening should be considered. This is effective in 70–80 per cent of patients with severe pain and the duration of relief is for up to six months. Malignant ascites can be managed as for gastric cancer, outlined previously. Chemotherapy is generally of little value in most patients with advanced pancreatic cancer.

LIVER AND BILIARY CANCER

All primary tumours of the liver and biliary system are rare; in contrast, hepatic metastases from other sites are a frequently encountered clinical problem.

Primary hepatocellular carcinoma (hepatoma) accounts for only 800 cancer registrations each year in the UK, although it is the most common malignancy throughout the world. In Britain 75–80 per cent of cases were associated with cirrhosis and present at a mean age of 55 years with fever, upper abdominal swelling, and discomfort. This is followed by jaundice and progressive failure of liver function. This malignancy can be associated with paraneoplastic problems: finger clubbing, hypercalcaemia, and erythrocytosis. The tumour usually spreads throughout the liver, but may be confined to one lobe at diagnosis. Venous spread occurs via the hepatic and portal veins to the vena cava; regional lymph node involvement and lung metastases are common.

A high (> 1000) serum level of alpha-fetoprotein is a diagnostic finding in many cases, particularly those with cirrhosis. Confirmation is by needle biopsy together with CT scanning, which defines the extent of regional spread.

For most patients with hepatocellular cancer the outlook is extremely poor: median survival from diagnosis being only 4–8 months. However, tumours that are confined to one lobe may be curable by lobectomy if the function of the remaining organ is adequate. In these patients, the five-year survival is up to 30 per cent, but most of those with cirrhosis will be unsuitable for the procedure. Liver transplantation has been successful in some patients.

Radiotherapy has little use because of the low tolerance of normal liver to radiation. Chemotherapy however can reduce liver size and discomfort; a good response is obtained in perhaps a quarter of people given adriamycin, 5-fluorouracil or mitomycin, and this is often associated with weight gain and marginal increase in survival. Regional perfusion of cytotoxic drugs via the hepatic artery may be used in the hope of increasing the response. New approaches include the use of monoclonal antibodies, labelled with radioiodine, which have a high specificity for hepatocellular carcinoma.

Tumour necrosis, which often leads to improvement in symptoms, can be produced by interference with tumour blood flow. This can be achieved by ligation of the hepatic artery at laparotomy or by transcutaneous embolization: fortunately the normal liver is supplied by the portal system.

Cholangiocarcionomas are mucin-secreting tumours. Those arising within the liver behave clinically as hepatocellular cancer while those at extrahepatic sites present with obstructive jaundice, similar to some pancreatic cancers. Occasionally they are discovered unexpecedly in cholecystectomy specimens.

Curative surgery entails a Whipples operation (pancreatoduodenectomy) for extrahepatic tumours and a partial hepatectomy may be possible for others arising within the liver. Radical radiotherapy may be appropriate in selected patients with small, well-defined tumours. Small volume external beam techniques sparing as much normal liver as possible are combined with intraluminal radiotherapy by cannulation of the biliary tree.

Surgical resection is possible in only 20 per cent and most patients with biliary cancer have a poor prognosis of less than six months. Palliation of obstructive jaundice can be achieved by a surgical by-pass procedure or by stenting of the distal bile ducts at endoscopy.

SECONDARY CANCER OF THE LIVER

Liver metastases arise frequently in gastrointestinal malignancies which are drained by the portal vein, but the organ is a common site of secondary spread from many other tumours, particularly lung and breast. This is sometimes the presenting feature of an occult primary malignancy the diagnosis is suggested by an enlarged liver, which is often hard and irregular. Liver function tests may be normal or reflect a mixture of cholestasis and parenchymal damage. Ultrasound scanning is more sensitive than isotope scintigraphy in demonstrating the lesions, which are frequently multiple. Histological proof is usually unnecessary in those cases with documented cancer elsewhere.

Patients with metastatic liver disease are incurable, with rare exceptions such as germ cell tumours, choriocarcinoma or some lymphomas—all of which are highly chemosensitive tumours. Surgical resection has occasionally been performed in highly selected patients, in whom tumour is confined to one lobe. This has lead to prolonged survival in a few patients with colorectal and carcinoid tumours. Most patients will die within a year of diagnosis and any active treatment must be given only after careful balancing of symptomatic benefit versus side-effects. Chemotherapy can be useful in patients who are still quite well and have responsive disease such as breast cancer, but often with minimal gain in duration of their survival. Low-dose irradiation of the liver is occasionally used for radiosensitive malignancy, for example breast cancer or lymphoma, where there is painful enlargement. Other invasive techniques include intra-arterial chemotherapy and embolization, but the majority of patients require simple, symptomatic care as discussed later in the chapter.

COLORECTAL CANCER

This the most common of all the gastrointestinal malignancies and fortunately is associated with a better prognosis. In England and Wales there are nearly 25 000 new cases annually but although up to 30 per cent survive five years, of whom many will be cured, colorectal cancer still causes more than 16 000 deaths each year.

Adenocarcinoma of the large bowel is the most frequently occurring malignacy after lung cancer in men, and after breast and lung cancer in women. Diet probably has a major part in its development, although the precise dietary modifications which would have an impact on these statistics remain uncertain. In families with polyposis, there is malignant change in a hyperproliferative mucosa, but these account for very few cases. Perhaps 12 per cent of all colonic cancers develop from sporadic adenomatous polyps and the risk of transformation increases with polyp size, while 40 per cent of villous adenomas undergo malignant change. Another well known association is with long-standing and extensive ulcerative colitis, with a marginally increased incidence in Crohn's disease.

Lymphoma and carcinoid tumours are also found in the large bowel but are extremely rare.

Direct spread of colonic cancer is by invasion through the bowel wall into the peritoneal cavity and adjacent viscera. Lymphatic dissemination occurs via the epi- and paracolic nodes and thence to perivascular nodes. As the colon is drained by the portal vein, liver metastases are common and are followed by involvement of the lung. Bone and cerebral deposits are not uncommon. Rectal tumours will eventually invade bladder, seminal vesicles, and prostate in men, or bladder and vagina in women; fistulae may develop in advanced disease. Cancer of the lower rectum has a different route of venous drainage; consequently liver metastases arise less frequently than with proximal tumours but local recurrence is a greater problem.

A total of 70 per cent of adenocarcinomas arise in the rectosigmoid colon. These cancers are likely to produce rectal bleeding and discharge; the stool becomes looser and the patient may have a persistent sensation of incomplete evacuation. It is said that three-quarters of all rectal tumours should be palpable on digital rectal examination; certainly early diagnosis depends upon prompt investigation of all rectal bleeding, even if there is an apparent innocuous source. Left-sided colonic tumours often cause a change in bowel habit, sometimes with obvious blood in the stool.

Episodes of distension and colicky pain may occur before unequivocal obstruction. More proximal tumours, especially those growing in the ascending colon, manifest themselves at a later stage. They may go undiagnosed until there is right iliac fossa pain with a mass or present as a surgical emergency when perforation supervenes. Others may present with anaemia or weight loss.

The investigation into altered bowel habit and blood loss includes visualization of the lower bowel and barium studies if the rectosigmoid appears normal. Candidates for elective surgery require screening for liver and lung metastases.

MANAGEMENT OF EARLY COLORECTAL CANCER

Tumours that are confined to the bowel wall are curable with surgery, which remains the standard treatment in all patients who are sufficiently fit for a radical procedure. Colonic cancer is resected together with a section of the mesentery and adjacent lymph nodes. This is usually performed at one operation, but two-stage procedures necessitating a temporary colostomy may be desirable where there is obstruction or any concern about the anastamosis.

An anterior resection is preferable for the patient with rectal cancer, who would like to avoid a permanent stoma, providing that this does not compromise the chance of cure. The use of stapling devices plus recognition that a narrower clearance margin may be adequate, has led to anterior resections being performed for tumours within 5–7 cm of the anal verge. Abdominoperineal resection is necessary for low rectal tumours; in these patients the procedure includes preoperative counselling and planned siting of the stoma.

The mortality from surgery at best is around 10 per cent, but rises with age, particularly in subjects over 70 years; the elderly are also more likely to have obstruction or perforation at presentation. Elective radical procedures are best confined to those cases where tumour has not spread beyond the lymphovascular pedicle adjacent to the involved section of bowel. It has been shown that those with further local spread may do as well with palliative resection. This applies particularly to frail patients of advanced age in whom even laser excision of early distal lesions may be acceptable.

Approximately 50 per cent of patients with colorectal cancer undergo radical surgery and 50 per cent of these are still alive at five years. The chance of cure is directly related to tumour stage: cancer confined to bowel wall (Dukes A) has a five-year survival of more than 70 per cent; beyond bowel (Dukes B) 50 per cent and with node involvement (Dukes C) 30 per cent. Due to the pattern of spread, the outcome in successfully resected colonic cancer is determined by the development of liver metastases.

In rectal cancer, although 60 per cent overall of operable disease is cured by surgery, failure is usually due to local recurrence rather than distant metastases. More than 40 per cent of node positive cases relapse with pelvic tumour. Efforts are being directed at improving local control, and, it is hoped, subsequent survival, by intensifying treatment for some patients.

It has been shown that postoperative radiotherapy to patients with Dukes stage B and C tumours reduces their risk of local recurrence; however the acute radiation reaction could interfere with healing of the wound and anastamosis. If patients are irradiated before their surgery (leaving an interval of four weeks), there should be the benefit of improved local control with less morbidity and there are advantages in prior reduction of the primary tumour mass where it is becoming fixed with borderline operability. It is of course important not to over-treat curable patients so the trials in progress are selecting those with operable disease but with peri-rectal spread.

Colorectal tumours show poor response rates to cytotoxic drugs; 5-fluorouracil is the most commonly employed but achieves a partial response in only 10–20 per cent which is enhanced by folinic acid. Attempts to improve survival in the poor prognostic groups, particularly those with Dukes C staging, have been disappointing. One new approach is the combination of chemotherapy with modifiers of the patient's own immune response such as levamisole, which is given as adjuvant treatment following surgery. Early results suggest that this may reduce the recurrence rate.

Often the first signs of relapse after colonic resection are related to the development of disseminated disease. Liver metastases produce loss of appetite, discomfort associated with organ enlargement, and eventually jaundice. Other intraperitoneal tumour masses may cause pain, ascites, and even obstruction. Lung metastases are the commonest problem outside the abdomen.

Rectal tumours are more likely to recur in the pelvis; this is usually within two years of surgery, although some low grade, slow-growing cancers may not manifest their recurrence for several years. Disease develops within the pre-sacral space and persistent ischial pain, later radiating as sciatica, is an early symptom. As progressive damage to sacral nerves develops, there is altered sensation in the corresponding dermatomes and urinary hesitancy leading to retention. Visible tumour may appear along the perineal scar while those patients who retained their rectum may complain of tenesmoid discomfort, bleeding or discharge. Recurrent tumour is often detectable on rectal or vaginal examination where this is possible; the diagnosis is confirmed by a pelvic CT scan.

MANAGEMENT OF ADVANCED COLORECTAL CANCER

Fit subjects with resectable primary disease are sometimes found to have distant spread, frequently to the liver, at laparotomy. As a group, these patients survive only 12 months on average, but resection of the bowel lesion is still justified to prevent subsequent obstruction or perforation. Where there is an apparently solitary liver deposit (which should be confirmed radiologically), resection of the liver metastasis as well as the primary can result in prolonged survival for a small number of patients.

In situations in which there is extensive or unresectable disease, a simple colostomy or by-pass procedure affords the best palliation for obstruction or fistulae.

Radiotherapy has an important role in the treatment of patients with rectal cancer who are inoperable at presentation or who develop postoperative pelvic recurrence. If the general condition of the patient is good and there is no distant spread, a prolonged course of treatment over several weeks is justified to achieve the best local tumour control. Patients who have had a previous abdominoperineal resection are spared the acute radiation proctitis which is the main side-effect of treatment. Radiotherapy alleviates pain in 50 per cent, bleeding in 75 per cent, and tenesmus/discharge in 30–40 per cent of patients treated. Useful palliation is still obtained from short courses in advanced cases where the patient's condition is poor; however, the anticipated life expectancy should be at least a few weeks for them to gain any benefit. Symptomatic metastatic disease, for example bone deposits, may be helped by radiotherapy, often by a single treatment session.

Chemotherapy is occasionally used in advanced symptomatic disease, for example single agent 5-fluorouracil which is administered orally or intravenously to patients with liver and lung metastases. It can also be instilled directly into the peritoneal cavity in cases with ascites. If infused through the hepatic artery, higher concentrations of the drug reach the liver and achieve a better response rate with hepatic metastases. No chemotherapy regimen offers any hope of cure and there is little convincing evidence that it confers any survival benefit.

MANAGEMENT OF COMMON SYMPTOMS IN ADVANCED GASTROINTESTINAL CANCER

Pain

Pain is present in 70 per cent of all patients with malignancy; most will have several coexistent pains and a key to successful pain control is careful consideration of the possible different causes. In gastrointestinal cancer, frequently occurring pains directly related to the tumour include:

(1) local invasion of adjacent tissues—paravertebral, abdominal wall;
(2) visceral pain—distension of the liver capsule, colic due to obstruction;
(3) nerve root compression or infiltration—retroperitoneal and pelvic tumour;
(4) bone metastases.

Much of cancer pain is chronic and often worsens with time as the disease progresses. This calls for the use of regular analgesics, titrated to the severity of the patient's pain. Fortunately, the early use of strong opioids for severe pain is now well established. Oral morphine, as instant-release tablets or solution, is used to control pain by regular four-hourly administration; some patients go through the night more easily if the bedtime dose is increased by 50 per cent. If a weak opioid (coproxamol, dihydrocodeine) has been used regularly, it is reasonable to commence 10 mg of morphine every four hours; the dose can be increased in increments of 50 per cent, every other day, to reach the optimum amount for pain control. Fortunately, there is no upper limit as long as the pain is clearly responding to morphine with no or minimal adverse effects. Reduced hepatic function has little effect on opioid requirements, but since the active metabolite, morphine-6-glucuronide, is renally excreted, any impairment of renal function necessitates slower titration. Eventually, the total 24-hour requirements can be converted to a twice-daily regimen using controlled release morphine preparations.

All patients should be reassured that mild to moderate drowsiness settles within 5–7 days at the same dose. It is kind to prescribe an antiemetic for the first 10 days to counteract the transient nausea experienced by some: haloperidol, 1.5–3 mg at night is effective. A regular laxative is essential; ideally this should combine a stool softener with stimulant (codanthramer or codanthrusate). A common error is to fail to titrate the laxative dose together with the opioid.

Diamorphine is used for parenteral administration, having greater solubility than morphine. This may be indicated when urgent pain relief is needed, or in patients unable to take drugs orally. The subcutaneous route gives less discomfort than the intra-muscular and is particularly useful for infusions. When converting from oral morphine, the 24-hour total is divided by three to find the amount of diamorphine required for the 24-hour infusion, which can be conveniently delivered with a syringe driver.

When there is poor pain control despite the use of regular analgesics titrated against the pain, the underlying causes should be reconsidered: it may be that the patients has pain which responds to opioids only partially or not at all, and a different approach is needed. Examples include colic, which responds to hyoscine butylbromide subcutaneously, and NSAIDs which are indicated in bone pain but may also help pain due to tumour infiltration at any site. High dose steroids, for example dexamethasone 16 mg daily, reduce peritumour oedema and they can be tried where the symptoms are related to a tumour mass, such as nerve root compression; they also relieve the discomfort associated with hepatomegaly.

Pain control can be particularly difficult in patients with retroperitoneal and pelvic tumour. The pre-sacral recurrence of a slowly-growing rectal carcinoma compresses and eventually damages nerves. After 1–3 months, the pain is associated with unpleasant dysaesthesia (deafferentation pain), often described by patients as burning, stabbing or numbness. This may respond to low-dose amitriptyline and/or carbamazepine, and the application of a TENS machine is helpful to some. In difficult cases the advice of an anaesthetist is valuable, as neurolytic procedures or spinal routes for drug administration may be appropriate. The use of coeliac blocks for pain with epigastic tumour has been mentioned previously.

Anorexia, nausea, and vomiting

Anorexia is perhaps the most common symptom in advanced cancer, especially in the terminal illness. At an earlier stage it is a source of great concern to both patient and family. There are a number of remediable causes: a sore mouth due to candida, gastritis, nausea for any reason, and also anxiety or depression. For other patients, corticosteroids remain the most effective treatment and the benefit is seen with dexamethasone 2–4 mg daily. Alternative, which sometimes help are megestrol acetate and cyproheptadine. It is helpful to suggest realistic goals, for example the enjoyment of one or two appetising snacks daily.

Nausea and vomiting cause much misery and as with pain control, it is important to consider the causes in each patient.

1. Chemical—drug induced (morphine, NSAIDS, antibiotics) metabolic (uraemia, toxaemia, hypercalcaemia).
2. Gastric compression or outlet obstruction.
3. Direct stimulation of vagal afferent nerves by intra-abdominal tumour, bowel distension (obstruction, constipation).

Anti-emetics have different pharmacological actions and successful treatment will depend upon the choice of appropriate drug or combination in addition to treating the underlying cause if possible. For example, emesis due to vagal stimulation often responds to cyclizine, which acts upon the vomiting centres. In contrast, the nausea, gastic stasis, and reflux associated with gastric compression is relieved by the combination of dimethicone with peripherally-acting drugs, such as domperidone.

Nausea caused by chemical stimulation will respond to low-dose haloperidol, which acts primarily on the chemoreceptor trigger zone and is particularly useful in treatment of opioid-induced nausea.

Intestinal obstruction

All obstructed patients require careful assessment, as a laparotomy should be considered unless they are terminally ill or thought to have extensive intraperitoneal disease with several levels of obstruction. These patients who are unsuitable for surgery, or indeed who might have declined further intervention, can often be kept comfortable without the use of intravenous fluids or nasogastric suction. Nausea and nearly all of the vomiting can be controlled using a subcutaneous infusion of cyclizine, combined if necessary with hyoscine butylbromide for colic. Diamorphine may be needed in addition for background pain. If the obstruction is not complete, a stool softener, such as docusate, may improve the situation. All patients are encouraged to continue regular oral fluids or even light diet if they wish. Most patients may be kept comfortable by this approach and it enables them to be managed at home for the duration of their terminal illness. A few will continue to have distressing vomits; where there is a high obstruction, a nasogastric tube to empty the stomach may be necessary. A venting gastrostomy is occasionally considered as an alternative where the anticipated survival is several weeks and other measures are unsuccessful.

PALLIATIVE CARE

The words 'I'm afraid there is nothing more to be done' have a terrible impact upon the cancer patient and his or her family. What is usually meant is that there is no specific anti-tumour therapy which could offer hope of cure or even temporary benefit at that point in time. Fortunately, this does not mean that there is no more treatment to help the individual, but all too often patients with advanced cancer are left to feel abandoned by the medical profession; they become isolated and assume that many distressing symptoms, particularly pain, are inevitable. The essence of good palliative care is in the effective control of symptoms, anticipation of clinical problems, and recognition of therapeutic opportunitites. Above all, it puts emphasisis on the quality of life for that individual.

The general practitioner and the primary care team play an essential role in the management of the patient with advanced disease, often with specialist nursing support at home, such as the Macmillan and Marie Curie nurses. The hospital specialties often continue their involvement, but with increasing ill health, out-patient attendance becomes onerous for the patient. Over the past 20 years, many hospices have been established within local communities to offer good terminal care. However, it is by no means necessary nor desirable for every patient to attend a hospice. More importantly, the hospice movement has led to the development of palliative medicine as a specialty, which is being used increasingly as a resource by doctors in hospitals and the community alike. Many palliative care units, whether based at a hospice, within a hospital or operating as a home-care team, offer advice on management of difficult problems and often admit patients for a short period for symptom control. This enables many to subsequently continue at home with their families as they would wish.

The essential goal in palliative care is to create an environment in which it is safe for the patient to express his or her distress. Such as atmosphere can be created at any bedside, whether home, hospital or hospice, providing there is empathy, knowledge, and commitment.

ACKNOWLEDGEMENT

The constructive advice of Dr C. Regnard was greatly appreciated in the preparation of this chapter.

FURTHER READING

Hope-Stone, H. F. (ed.) (1988). *Radiotherapy in clinical practice*. Butterworth, Oxford.

Magrath, I. (ed.) (1989). *New directions in cancer treatment*. Springer-Verlag, Berlin.

Cuschieri, A., Giles, G. R., and Moosa, A. R. (1988). *Essential surgical practice*. Wright, Bristol.

Twycross, R. and Lack, S. (1986). *Control of alimentary symptoms in far advanced cancer*. Churchill Livingstone, London.

Sikora, K. and Halnan, K. E. (1990). *Treatment of cancer*. Chapman and Hall, London.

13 Surgery of the gastro-intestinal tract

Greg Rubin and Brendan Devlin

The past decade has seen immense changes in the surgical management of gastrointestinal disease. Elective surgery for peptic ulceration is now almost defunct, and it may not be long before open cholecystectomy follows suit. Stapling instruments have transformed colorectal surgery, allowing sphincter-saving procedures to be carried out in more patients with rectal cancer. The same drive to preserve sphincter function in the surgical treatment of ulcerative colitis has seen the development of the ileal reservoir.

This chapter does not catalogue the whole panoply of gastrointestinal surgery, but rather concentrates on selected conditions of importance to general practitioners. These have been chosen because we commonly make decisions on surgical management, as in the referral of patients with gallstones for cholecystectomy, or because surgical treatment gives rise to complications which can be long-term or difficult to manage, as with stomas or duodenal ulcer surgery.

GASTRO-OESOPHAGEAL REFLUX

Gastro-oesophageal reflux disease (GORD) is now, for reasons that are unclear, the most common upper gastrointestinal problem encountered by physicians. It may be that we as general practitioners are becoming more discriminatory as to the types of dyspepsia, recognizing GORD as a distinct entity. At the same time, new, specific, and effective drugs, such as omeprazole and cisapride, have added significantly to our therapeutic options for this condition. Indeed, surgical treatment of GORD is very much the Cinderella option, unloved and often forgotten, tarnished by a reputation for unpleasant, and sometimes serious, side-effects. And yet failure to consider anti-reflux surgery soon enough risks the development of irreversible complications, such as stenosis, Barrett's oesophagus or malignant transformation.

Indications for surgery

Failure of medical treatment is the most common reason for surgery, accounting for more than 85 per cent of all cases. Failure is usually due to the anti-reflux barrier being defective to the point where serious reflux continues despite therapy. It can be defined as the persistence of intractable symptoms after six months' treatment with an H_2-receptor antagonist or proton pump inhibitor. The diagnosis should be confirmed by endoscopy, together with pH monitoring and oesophageal manometry if any doubts exist.

Complications of gastro-oesophageal reflux, peptic stricture, haemorrhage, and respiratory complications account for the remainder of surgical interventions. Up to a fifth of patients with reflux may have significant respiratory problems due to repeated aspiration of gastric contents, sometimes leading to pulmonary fibrosis. A link between GORD and asthma has also been postulated.

Although hospital-based studies suggest that up to 60 per cent of patients referred with GORD undergo surgery, they apply to highly selected groups wholly unrepresentative of the full spectrum of reflux disease seen in general practice.

Surgical techniques

The aim of surgery is to restore the anti-reflux barrier by maintaining the pressure gradient between the stomach and the lower oesophagus.

Anatomical repairs (Allison's repair, gastropexy) produce disappointing results and have largely been abandoned in favour of anti-reflux procedures. The best known of these is the Nissen fundoplication.

The Nissen operation uses an abdominal approach, the gastric fundus being wrapped as a cuff around the lower oesophagus or upper stomach, thereby preventing reflux of gastric contents.

Long-term outcome

The success of anti-reflux surgery is highly operator-dependent. Although operative mortality is less than 0.5 per cent, surgical failure is difficult to correct by a second operation and patients should therefore only be referred to centres with a special interest and surgical skill in anti-reflux surgery.

Dysphagia, hypercontinence, and 'gas bloat' are the most common postoperative complications of fundoplication.

Dysphagia can occur in up to 50 per cent of patients undergoing fundoplication, but is usually mild and transient, resolving within three weeks. After six months only 5 per cent of patients will have dysphagia, falling to 2 per cent after 12 months.

Hypercontinence is a result of the complete elimination of reflux achieved by surgical correction of gastro-oesophageal sphincter insufficiency. Belching and vomiting become very difficult or even impossible.

This is compounded by the habit some patients with reflux disease have of swallowing air to improve acid clearance from the oesophagus. This habit remains after surgery, but air cannot now be regurgitated and collects in the gut, distending the stomach and small intestine and making the patient feel replete—hence the term gas bloat. Gas bloat and hypercontinence are generally mild and tend to disappear with time. Two per cent of patients have disabling symptoms requiring revisional surgery.

Failure to relieve reflux symptoms is most commonly caused by disruption of the fundal wrap or by its distal migration—the 'slipped' Nissen. Recurrent symptoms due to these causes will often become apparent within the first post-operative year.

The Angelchik prosthesis is a procedure now discredited because of its high complication rate. After 12 months, 30 per cent of patients still had mild dysphagia, while a further 10 per cent had moderate to severe dysphagia requiring removal of the prosthesis. The prosthesis may also require removal because of migration or erosion into the oesophagus or stomach. Upward movement causes severe dysphagia, movement downwards over the stomach results in early satiety and vomiting.

DUODENAL ULCER

Although hospital admissions for duodenal ulcer steadily declined in the 1960s and 1970s, the introduction of H_2-receptor antagonists in 1977 accelerated this trend dramatically through the 1980s. At the same time, the causes of admission for duodenal ulcer disease changed. Elective surgery for duodenal ulcer has become increasingly uncommon, but emergency admission for haemorrhage or perforation remains unchanged, though an increasing proportion of patients are elderly women. The mortality rate from these two complications is 10–15 per cent and has not been reduced by the use of H_2-receptor antagonists. There are currently 4500 deaths per year in England and Wales from haemorrhage and perforation, the mean age of death being 71 years.

Surgical management of duodenal ulceration is indicated for:

(1) perforation;
(2) severe haemorrhage;
(3) pyloric stenosis;
(4) failure of medical treatment.

The first three indications present little difficulty in definition, but the fourth has been continuously refined through extended experience with H_2-receptor antagonists and, more recently, with proton pump inhibitors.

At present, conservative management is deemed to have failed in the following situations:

(1) medical treatment fails to heal the ulcer;
(2) the patient frequently relapses on maintenance therapy;
(3) the patient relapses early after three or more full courses of ulcer healing treatment.

In assessing the need for surgery the duration and severity of symptoms must also be carefully assessed to establish the effect of the disease on quality of life. Useful indicators in this respect are night waking, loss of time from work, and hospital admissions.

A case can also be argued for special consideration of patients with established ulcer disease who experience relapses around the age of 50 years. At this age there is a 25 per cent risk of bleeding and a 10 per cent risk of perforation, and these risks increase over subsequent decades. The mortality rate for both complications is 10 per cent. Active surgical management in this age group is relatively safe and could significantly reduce this mortality rate.

Surgery for duodenal ulcer was initially orientated towards curing the ulcer and preventing relapse. As a result, a number of variations on partial resection of the stomach with or without vagotomy were developed. These included:

(1) partial gastrectomy with gastroduodenal anastomosis (Billroth I);
(2) partial gastrectomy with gastrojejunal anastomosis (Billroth II);
(3) truncal vagotomy and antrectomy with gastroduodenal anastomosis;
(4) truncal vagotomy and gastrojejunostomy;
(5) truncal vagotomy and pyloroplasty.

It became apparent that these procedures had a significant operative mortality (1 per cent) and serious post-operative problems, such as dumping, biliary gastritis, and metabolic changes. Highly selective vagotomy (partial vagotomy, proximal gastric vagotomy) has a mortality rate of 0.3 per cent and avoids these complications, and has therefore gained increasing favour. Although there is an ulcer recurrence rate after 10 years of 15 per cent, it is the elective procedure of choice, since recurrent ulcers are considerably easier to treat than the side-effects of gastrectomy or drainage.

Previous surgical practice has, however, left a legacy of long-term post-operative problems. Some centres still run out-patient clinics to follow up patients after gastric surgery, though the trend is to discharge responsibility for this to the general practitioner. An awareness of the problems that may be encountered is therefore valuable in managing these patients.

Common problems

Dysphagia

Dysphagia occurs in 20 per cent of patients following vagotomy. It is probably due to surgical trauma and oedema around the oesophagus. Most cases resolve over a few weeks with a fluid diet. Occasionally, endoscopy and dilatation may be necessary if dysphagia is persistent.

Small stomach syndrome

This occurs after extensive gastric resection and presents with early satiety, epigastric pain and fullness and nausea and vomiting, together with weight loss. Treatment includes nutritional advice and small frequent meals. Some patients require the construction of a jejunal pouch and restoration of duodenal continuity—a procedure of variable benefit.

Early dumping

This is the most common side-effect of gastric surgery. Its symptoms are shown in Table 13.1. It occurs because pyloric function is lost or impaired and is caused by the rapid gastric emptying of hyperosmolar contents from the stomach into the small intestine. It occurs during or immediately after a meal and postulated mechanisms include:

(1) distension of the jejunum stimulating autonomic reflexes;
(2) systemic hypovolaemia due to fluid shift into the bowel in response to hypertonic contents;
(3) release of vaso-active regulatory peptides.

Treatment consists principally of dietary manipulation. Meals should be small and frequent, and not accompanied by fluids. Food should be high in fibre and low in carbohydrate to reduce the osmotic load.

There is no specific medical treatment, though somatostatin and its

Table 13.1 *Symptoms of early dumping syndrome*

Systemic	Abdominal
Sweating	Fullness
Faintness	Nausea
Palpitations	Vomiting
Headaches	Epigastric pain
Flushing	Diarrhoea
Pallor	

analogue octreotide have been found to be useful in some studies. Surgical treatment is indicated in about 5 per cent of patients for whom symptoms are severe and intractable and last more than 1–2 years. The aim is to slow gastric emptying and the interposition of an isoperistaltic jejunal segment is probably the most effective procedure.

Enterogastric reflux

Enterogastric reflux, or biliary gastritis, occurs in up to 20 per cent of patients after partial gastrectomy, and up to 7 per cent after highly selective vagotomy. Loss of the antro-pyloric reflux barrier allows reflux of upper intestinal secretions, especially bile, into the stomach. This produces symptoms of pain, vomiting, and weight loss. The pain is constant, made worse by food and not relieved by antacids.

Endoscopy shows diffuse gastritis with bile staining and also serves to exclude alternative diagnoses, such as recurrent ulceration or reflux oesophagitis. It typically comes on before breakfast and is relieved by vomiting.

Medical treatment is helpful in mild cases. Cholestyramine will bind bile salts, sucralfate is a mucosal protective agent, metoclopramide and cisapride promote gastric emptying.

The most common surgical treatment of enterogastric reflux is Roux en Y diversion. This relieves symptoms in 80 per cent of patients, but they must subsequently take H_2-receptor antagonists indefinitely to prevent marginal ulceration.

Diarrhoea

Diarrhoea is most common after truncal vagotomy and drainage, affecting 30 per cent of patients, and occurs in less than 10 per cent of patients undergoing highly selective vagotomy. It commonly occurs within 1–2 hours of meals, but may sometimes be severe and intractable with marked urgency, seriously impairing the quality of life. The postulated causes include rapid gastric emptying and rapid intestinal transit. Typical post-prandial symptoms need no further investigation, but patients with severe symptoms should be assessed to exclude other causes, such as coeliac disease or blind loop syndrome.

The dietary manipulation used to help dumping is also effective for diarrhoea. Loperamide or codeine phosphate can also be given. Further surgery has nothing to offer.

Recurrent ulceration

This has been the subject of extensive study. After 10 years the recurrence rate for highly selective vagotomy is 15 per cent, for vagotomy and drainage 10 per cent, and for Billroth II resection 5 per cent. The high recurrence rate after highly selective vagotomy is outweighed by the favourable response of recurrent ulcers to medical treatment and the low incidence of dumping and diarrhoea with this procedure. Most recurrent ulcers are due to inadequate surgery, particularly incomplete vagotomy. Drugs, especially NSAIDs, alcohol, and smoking are also causative factors. Recurrent ulceration usually causes the patients their pre-operative symptoms but can be symptomless.

Endoscopy is essential for diagnosis since barium meal may miss 50 per cent of recurrent ulcers.

Recurrent ulcers usually respond to treatment with H_2-receptor antagon-ists or omeprazole. Re-operation, which is difficult and has a higher mortality, is determined by the original operation but usually consists of revagotomy and antrectomy, since vagotomy without resection has a high ulcer recurrence rate.

Metabolic problems

These are common several years after surgery, but are rarely severe. Weight loss may occur, though the incidence of this complication varies widely between studies. It is usually due to malnutrition, food intake having been reduced to try to avoid symptoms such as pain, dumping, and diarrhoea.

Malabsorption is a rare cause of weight loss after gastric surgery.

Most patients develop mild iron deficiency anaemia 5–10 years after gastrectomy, though levels below 10 g/dl are unusual. It rarely occurs after vagotomy alone. Factors which contribute to iron deficiency anaemia include reduced dietary intake, the loss of H^+ ions to convert ferric to ferrous iron, chronic blood loss due to stomal gastritis, and reduced absorption due to faster small bowel transit or duodenal bypass (Billroth II).

Vitamin B_{12} deficiency may also contribute to anaemia. This can occur either because of poor dietary intake, or because rapid gastric emptying does not allow sufficient time for the B_{12}—intrinsic factor complex to form. Treatment with B_{12} or folate supplements should be long-term, as relapses otherwise occur.

Disturbances of calcium metabolism are found in 20 per cent of patients 10 years after gastric resection, but are rarely seen after vagotomy. They are principally related to a reduced intake of calcium and vitamin D but rarely give rise to symptoms such as bone fractures or osteomalacia.

Long-term follow-up of patients after any gastric resection or drainage procedure should therefore include estimation of haemoglobin, B_{12}, folate, serum iron, and iron binding capacity. Estimation of calcium, phosphate and alkaline phosphatase is also appropriate for those who have undergone gastric resection, but not for those who merely had a drainage procedure. Such follow-up is not necessary for patients who have undergone highly selective vagotomy.

Rare problems

Late dumping

This occurs 2–3 hours after a meal and is due to hypoglycaemia. It presents as sweating, palpitations, weakness, and confusion, and is resolved by taking sugar.

Cancer risk

The risk of cancer is increased after gastric resection for peptic ulcer. An increase in mortality only occurs after the first post-operative 15 years and is multi-organ, suggesting the production in the stomach of circulating carcinogen with a long latency period. The risk of gastric cancer 20 years after gastric surgery is 4.5 × normal. It is also increased for other sites, notably the biliary tract (× 9.1), bronchus (× 3.9), and pancreas (× 4). The risk of cancer for all sites is increased threefold.

Other rare complications of gastric surgery include:

(1) reflux oesophagitis;
(2) phytobezoars;
(3) cholelithiasis;
(4) afferent loop syndrome.

GALLSTONES

Gallstones increase in frequency with age. They are present in 17 per cent of all adults and in 30 per cent of all 80-year-old women. They are more common in multiparous women and the obese, and are predisposed to by ileal resection and possibly vagotomy. For many years, regardless of the nature of symptoms attributed to them, their type or position, the treatment of gallstones was open cholecystectomy, and in 1986 40 000 cholecystectomies were performed in England and Wales. The past decade, however, has seen a huge increase in the range of alternative treatments. Gallstones can now be dissolved or fragmented *in-situ*; they can be removed from the gall-bladder with a percutaneous approach, or from the common bile duct using an endoscope. The most recent development, laparoscopic cholecystectomy, may yet prove to be the most revolutionary of all.

An important lesson of recent years has been the importance of careful selection of patients for surgery, as listed below.

1. Emergency cholecystectomy—biliary peritonitis; acute cholecystitis failing to settle on conservative treatment.
2. Early cholecystectomy (within 7 days)—acute cholecystitis; acalculous cholecystitis; acute pancreatitis due to gallstones.
3. Elective cholecystectomy—gallstones causing chronic cholecystitis or recurrent biliary colic.

Patients with prolonged attacks of right upper quadrant pain are more likely to have continued pain after cholecystectomy and should be carefully assessed for alternative causes. Particular caution should be exercised in the patient with gall-bladder dyspepsia. Symptoms of epigastric discomfort, flatulence, nausea, and fat intolerance are common and may be related to delayed gastric emptying or oesophageal reflux, even if gallstones have been demonstrated. Such dyspepsia has been shown to be equally common in patients with and without gallstones. Patients with gallstones and biliary pain who also complain of dyspepsia do well after cholecystectomy in terms of dyspepsia relief, but patients with gallstones selected for cholecystectomy because of dyspepsia alone do badly, 50 per cent relapsing within two years.

The asymptomatic or 'silent' gallstone presents an increasingly common problem. The widespread use of ultrasonography in particular has led to more frequent incidental detection. Why stones become symptomatic, and when, is less clear. It may depend on chance movement of stones and their impaction in the cystic duct on passage into the common bile duct. The concept of a latent period between stone formation and symptom onset is disputed, though one small study using carbon dating concluded that there is a mean delay of eight years between the two events. Since 90 per cent of patients with silent gallstones will remain asymptomatic, and given the low mortality of early operative intervention when symptoms arise, the consensus of surgical opinion is that cholecystectomy is not indicated in these patients.

There are three situations, however, in which elective cholecystectomy for silent gallstones should be considered. Diabetic patients with asymptomatic gallstones are more likely to develop acute cholecystitis than non-diabetics. Diabetic patients also have higher morbidity and mortality rates following emergency surgery, probably because of a higher incidence of coincidental disease.

Prophylactic cholecystectomy should therefore be seriously considered for diabetic patients with silent stones, indeed screening of adult patients with diabetes may be desirable.

Cholecystectomy should also be considered if gallstones are found at laparotomy for an unrelated condition, since post-operative cholecystitis is a well-recognized entity. Some surgeons now urge screening for gallstones in all patients about to undergo major abdominal surgery.

Gall-bladder cancer has long been cited, erroneously, as a reason for cholecystectomy for asymptomatic stones. This tumour has an extremely poor prognosis but only occurs in 2 per cent of patients with stones. In the 'porcelain' or calcified gallbladder, however, the incidence rises to between 20 and 60 per cent, and cholecystectomy is recommended in this instance.

Operative techniques

Open cholecystectomy

The most common treatment for gallstones is still open cholecystectomy, together with exploration of the common bile duct should an operative cholangiogram be abnormal. It is an operation with a low mortality rate, figures of 0.25 per cent having been reported. Post-operative complications, which include wound sepsis, venous thrombosis, and bile duct injury, are usually the result of faulty operative technique. Pain from the upper abdominal scar tends to 'splint' the chest and diaphragm, and chest infections are a common complication.

Endoscopic sphincterotomy

The primary treatment for bile duct stones, whether elective or as an emergency, is now endoscopic sphincterotomy. An open surgical approach is nowadays reserved for those patients who need a cholecystectomy and those in whom endoscopic treatment has failed. Though most stones less than 1 cm in diameter will eventually pass spontaneously after sphincterotomy, many endoscopists prefer to extract the stones directly, thereby avoiding the risks of impaction, cholangitis or pancreatitis. Success rates of 95 per cent have been achieved for sphincterotomy, with successful stone extraction in at least 90 per cent. There is a morbidity rate of 10 per cent and mortality of 1 per cent. The procedure is done under sedation and patients are usually discharged the following day.

Lithotripsy

Much interest has centred in recent years on the use of extra-corporeal shock wave lithotripsy in treating gallstones. This is a procedure which can be carried out under sedation with a hospital stay of 2–4 days. Newer techniques can even be used on an out-patient basis.

The criteria for selection for this treatment, however, make it one of limited value. The patient must have a radiolucent stone or stones of a minimum size and maximum number within a functioning gall-bladder. They must also take oral dissolution therapy for at least three and up to 12 months afterwards.

Percutaneous cholecystolithotomy

This is an alternative method of stone extraction, avoiding cholecystectomy, which is suitable for those patients for whom lithotripsy is not appropriate. The gall-bladder is percutaneously cannulated under ultrasound guidance at two separate points. The stones are extracted by flushing with saline, larger stones being fragmented before removal.

Patients stay in hospital for 3–4 days on external biliary drainage and need to take dissolution therapy for six weeks afterwards. Success rates of 85 per cent have been reported.

Laparoscopic cholecystectomy

One advance above all others has revolutionized the treatment of gallstones. Laparoscopic cholecystectomy allows removal of both stones and gall-bladder, thereby avoiding recurrence. It has major advantages over standard cholecystectomy in respect of length of hospital stay, post-operative pain, return to work and cosmetic appearance. The technique uses a viewing laparoscope with a television camera at the eyepiece, passed through a port at the umbilicus. Three operating ports are then created, the principal one being sited below the xiphoid process. The cystic duct and artery are clipped and divided. The gall-bladder is then dissected using diathermy or a laser. An important feature of the dissection is the ability to obtain meticulous hemostasis. The gall-bladder can then be removed intact through the umbilicus, large stones being crushed *in-situ* before removal.

Up to 90 per cent of patients currently undergoing standard chole-cystectomy may be eligible for this procedure. Early exclusion criteria included acute cholecystitis, common bile duct stones, obesity, and previous abdominal surgery. As experience has been gained, so previous abdominal surgery has posed less of a problem. Common bile duct stones can be dealt with by endoscopic sphincterotomy either before or after laporoscopic cholecystectomy, though laparoscopic methods for exploring the common bile duct are now being perfected.

Although laparoscopic cholecystectomy takes longer than open cholecystectomy—between 1 and 2 hours—post-operative pain is minimal and 70 per cent of patients can be discharged within 24 hours. More than 90 per cent can resume normal activities by the seventh post-operative day.

Late complications

Late complications of cholecystectomy can include recurrent stones, biliary stricture, and post-cholecystectomy symptoms. The use of operative cholangiography to view the biliary ducts has reduced the incidence of recurrent stones significantly, most of which had been overlooked in the first operation. Stones may form *de novo* in a dilated common bile duct. Presenting symptoms include cholangitis, jaundice or recurrent pancreatitis. Accurate visualization using percutaneous transhepatic cholangiography (PTC) or endoscopic retrograde cholangio-pancreatography (ERCP) is necessary for diagnosis. Treatment may be by endoscopic sphincterotomy and stone extraction or, if the ducts are grossly dilated, surgical re-exploration, stone extraction, and choledochoduodenostomy.

Post-operative biliary stricture caused by ductal injury occurs once in every 500 cases of cholecystectomy. It may present months or even years later, usually with recurrent jaundice and cholangitis. Percutaneous transhepatic cholangiography will provide an accurate diagnosis. Surgical repair is the treatment of choice and the mortality for uncomplicated strictures is less than 1 per cent. Patients with a bile duct injury should be followed up with clinical assessment and liver function tests. Recurrent symptoms or deterioration in liver function would indicate the need for further investigation.

Post-cholecystectomy symptoms are the most common problem encountered. One third of patients continue to experience pain after cholecystectomy, whilst 20–50 per cent will continue to complain of dyspepsia. These apparently poor results are largely due to an operation being performed for symptoms that were not due to gallstones in the first instance, and emphasize the importance of careful selection of patients for cholecystectomy.

Assessment of patients with post-cholecystectomy symptoms requires upper gastrointestinal endoscopy to exclude gastric or duodenal ulceration, and ERCP to demonstrate the biliary and pancreatic ductal systems. Coincidental upper gastrointestinal pathology is more likely in those patients presenting with dyspepsia, even when previous investigations have been normal. The most common findings are reflux oesophagitis, hiatus hernia or peptic ulceration. Patients presenting with jaundice, cholangitis or pancreatitis usually have a demonstrable abnormality on ERCP. Pancreatic disease may have passed unnoticed at the time of the original surgery.

INFLAMMATORY BOWEL DISEASE

A third of patients with total ulcerative colitis and 55 per cent of those with colonic Crohn's disease will require surgery within five years of disease onset.

Ulcerative colitis treated by proctocolectomy and ileostomy has a 100 per cent cure rate; the same procedure done for colonic Crohn's disease carries a 15 per cent recurrence at 15 years. These bland figures conceal a major burden of physical and psychological trauma, against which can be set the considerable improvement in well-being that surgery for chronic disease can achieve. As a result, surgeons have striven to develop procedures that improve the post-operative quality of life, the continent ileostomy and the Parks pouch being notable examples.

In acute ulcerative colitis, surgery is indicated for deteriorating toxic megacolon and for fulminating colitis not responding to medical treatment. Surgery for chronic disease should be considered when there is recurrent or continuous disease creating constant symptoms that fail to respond to medical treatment.

Operative techniques

Sub-total colectomy with ileostomy

This is the procedure of choice for acute ulcerative colitis, bringing out the distal colon as a mucous fistula. This deals with the acute problem but preserves the option of subsequent restorative surgery.

The choice of surgical procedure for patients with chronic ulcerative colitis lies between total colectomy with ileo-rectal anastomosis and a proctocolectomy with or without reservoir. Total colectomy with ileorectal anastomosis is not widely practised. Although it leaves the anal sphincter unchanged and avoids a stoma, it is not a curative procedure; the risk of subsequent proctectomy for cancer or recurrent disease ranges from 13 to 40 per cent, demanding annual sigmoidoscopy and rectal biopsies.

Proctocolectomy with Brooke ileostomy

This has been the standard treatment for many years. It is the fastest and safest operation, allows the earliest return to work, and has the least risk of complications. An ileostomy, however, has enormous psychological drawbacks in terms of alteration of body image and loss of sphincter control, together with the physical effects of an alteration in fluid balance.

The Koch Pouch

This was an early modification to this procedure. It comprises the construction of a pouch from the ileum into which the terminal ileum is invaginated to produce a one-way valve. This reservoir must be emptied 3–4 times a day by catheterization. It has the advantage of not requiring appliances, but valve failure leads to a need for corrective surgery in more than 40 per cent of patients and there is an overall continence rate of only 80 per cent. This option appeals to patients who have a failed ileo-anal reservoir or who are unhappy with the standard ileostomy and want to change it to this continent alternative.

The ileal pouch

This is an ileal reservoir with ileoanal anastomosis, first described in 1978. The original method has since been considerably modified, reducing the size of rectal cuff and increasing the pouch volume in the process. The use of surgical staplers has also simplified this type of surgery. As a result, patients undergoing this procedure can expect to be continent most of the time, have six bowel actions by day and one by night, delay defecation for 30 minutes and retain normal bladder and sexual function. The principal disadvantage is that 2–3 centimetres of rectal mucosa remain. The risk of neoplastic change is relatively small, however, and surveillance is easy.

The formation of an ileal pouch is not an option in the treatment of Crohn's colitis because of the risk of small bowel recurrence within the pouch. The choice of treatment for this condition lies between resection and total proctocolectomy with excision of the anus.

Ileo-rectal anastomosis

This is suitable for patients with Crohn's colitis in whom the rectum and anus are spared. Even then 40 per cent will need a second operation for recurrent disease. The ileum is invariably involved at this stage and revisional surgery usually involves ileal resection and total proctectomy. Even after total proctocolectomy as a primary procedure, 20 per cent of patients will require revisional surgery—namely ileal resection.

Long-term complications

Stomas

Although the preservation of continence by formation of an ileal pouch is increasingly the procedure of choice, thereby reducing the number of new ileostomies formed each year, there remain approximately 10 000 ileostomates in the UK today. They are at risk of a wide range of physical, social, and psychological problems, many of which are common to patients with a colostomy and are dealt with later in the chapter.

Of the physical problems specific to the ileostomate, that of chronic but usually symptomless salt and water depletion is the most important. This becomes clinically relevant in coincidental illnesses when fluid loss is increased, such as gastroenteritis. The incidence of urolithiasis is also higher due to low urinary pH, low urine output, and high plasma uric acid. There is an increased risk of cholelithiasis, particularly amongst those ileostomates whose primary pathology is Crohn's disease. Recurrent intestinal obstruction is a problem in all patients who undergo panproctocolectomy, the estimated annual incidence being 15 per cent.

Social activities are restricted after stoma surgery. Patients exert conscious control over the range and type of their social participation. Eighty per cent of ileostomates consider they lead a normal social life, although 17 per cent give up some sporting activity, while the remaining 20 per cent are limited by a fear of problems such as inappropriate stoma function or lack of suitable bathroom facilities.

Return to work is achieved by 90 per cent of ileostomates, though some are restricted by poor sanitary arrangements in the workplace or a hot working environment.

Body image changes as a result of the loss of the anus and creation of a stoma. Ostomates may see themselves as weak and vulnerable with feelings of shame, degradation, and fear of rejection. They may grieve for their loss—their grief reaction being associated with a sensation of phantom rectum. Although female ileostomates show good psychological adaptation after surgery, their male counterparts show considerably increased introversion and aggressiveness.

Sexual function may be impaired by physical or psychological causes. Indeed the two may be interrelated in male sexual dysfunction, the incidence of which may be as high as 30 per cent. There is a lower postoperative marriage rate in female ileostomates. Swedish women ileostomates have fewer extra-marital experiences than controls. Homosexuals can experience severe psychosexual problems after rectal excision and need careful counselling. Intercourse via the stoma may be attempted. This is dangerous and patients should be advised of the risk.

Contraception after stoma surgery presents a number of difficulties. Oral contraceptives may not be adequately absorbed. The distorted pelvic anatomy makes the use of an intrauterine contraceptive device or diaphragm difficult. Condoms or depot contraception are the best options. Female sterilization is difficult because of pelvic adhesions and the danger to loops of intestine.

Pouches

Surgical complications associated with pouches are highly operator dependent and this surgery is best performed in centres with a substantial body of existing and ongoing experience.

Anal sphincter tone is affected by the trans-anal dissection required during pouch formation and ileo-anal anastomosis. Many patients have a mucoid anal leakage at night to begin with, though most improve over the first 12 months.

Pouch failure requiring excision occurs in 10 per cent of patients and is most often due to fistulae, sepsis, stenosis or pouchitis.

Pouchitis can be a significant problem, presenting with fever and watery diarrhoea and being associated with non-specific mucosal inflammation. Its aetiology is unknown, but symptoms often resolve with metronidazole. Although usually limited it can sometimes be so persistent or unresponsive as to require removal of the pouch and formation of a standard ileostomy.

Sexual and bladder dysfunction are much less likely than with ileostomy because of the less extensive pelvic dissection required.

COLORECTAL CANCER

Colorectal cancer has an incidence of 38 per 100 000 in England and Wales and accounts for almost 17 000 deaths per year in the UK, a figure exceeded only by deaths from carcinoma of the bronchus. Its surgical treatment has undergone a revolution in the past decade through the introduction of stapling instruments. These devices, which permit more accurate anastomosis and a smaller tumour-free margin, have allowed more patients to be treated by sphincter-saving resection.

One third of rectosigmoid cancers are incurable due to advanced local/regional and distant disease. The increasing longevity of the population has also meant that more diagnoses of rectal cancer are being made in patients either unfit to withstand 'curative' surgery or with disseminated disease. As a result, techniques of local treatment have been developed to achieve palliative relief of bleeding, tenesmus, and obstructive symptoms.

Palliative surgical resection

This carries a morbidity of up to 50 per cent, and as high as 17 per cent mortality. It requires prolonged recovery in what may only be a short survival period, and may require a permanent colostomy as well.

Laser resection

Resection using an Nd-YAG laser, can produce effective palliation with low morbidity on a day case or short-stay basis. The laser beam is delivered down an optical fibre via a flexible sigmoidoscope to coagulate and vaporize the tumour surface. Symptomatic improvement occurs after 1–3 treatments in more than 80 per cent of patients. Treatment is repeated every 6–8 weeks, rather than waiting for symptom recurrence. The technique is better at palliating tenesmus and discharge than relieving obstruction, and may not help low rectal lesions where the anal sphincter is disturbed. It does not help pain due to pelvic wall infiltration.

Radiotherapy

Radiotherapy is helpful for 50 per cent of patients with tenesmus or discharge. Unfortunately it is of short-lived benefit, has multiple complications, and may require a defunctioning colostomy.

Photodynamic therapy

This is the destruction of tissue by an exogenous cytotoxic chemical which is activated by light. For colorectal tumours this is done using a dye laser via the colonoscope. The main disadvantage of this therapy is that tumour destruction is limited by penetration of the laser light. This makes it most effective in patients with small tumours or those with residual areas of tumour after initial debulking by surgical or laser therapy.

There remain 5000 patients per year in the UK who have their colorectal cancer treated by abdomino-perineal resection with permanent end colostomy and there are approximately 100 000 patients with a colostomy in the UK today. As with ileostomy, the range of morbidity after the formation of a colostomy is remarkable for its spread across the physical, social, and psychological spectrum. A composite measure of colostomy problems, for example, showed that 90 per cent of patients experience one or more problems with stoma management. Four-fifths of colostomates also have at least one chronic ailment, the most common being rheumatoid arthritis and rheumatism. One-sixth are disabled, a feature associated with increasing age and female sex.

Physical recovery

The formation of a colostomy occurs as part of an extensive surgical procedure performed on an often debilitated patient. Physical recovery takes three months or more and is influenced by the extent of the underlying disease and its subsequent course.

Complications that may become apparent at this stage include ischaemia, retraction or prolapse, stenosis and herniation. Retraction and prolapse often require surgical revision. Para-stomal herniation is common, occurring in 20 per cent of colostomates.

Bleeding from a colostomy should always be investigated. Five per cent of colorectal cancer patients develop a metachronous cancer, which may present with bleeding or with alteration in stoma habit. Bleeding may also occur from cancer on the colostomy arising by lymphatic spread or by cancer colonization.

Stoma management

Many of the problems of stoma management are common to both ileostomates and colostomates and are therefore dealt with together.

Dietary modification

Dietary modification, sometimes to a severe degree, is used by 50 per cent of ostomates in an effort to regulate stoma function. Many others restrict certain foods because of their effects on stool consistency, odour or flatus. Only a small range of foodstuffs, notably green vegetables and onions, produce symptoms in a significant proportion of patients. Dietary items that appear to cause problems should be tried at least on three separate occasions before being eliminated.

Air travel

This poses particular problems for the ostomate, since the appliance fills with gas as height is gained and barometric pressure falls. Although flatus filters help circumvent this, spare equipment should always be carried in the hand baggage.

Medication

Medication to regulate stoma function is used regularly by a quarter of ostomates and occasionally by a further quarter. There is, however, little correlation between stoma function and either diet or regular medication.

Irrigation

Though widely practised in the USA, irrigation is most unusual in the UK despite its now accepted safety. Most ostomates manage their stoma by means of a bag, although a minority with a colostomy can manage with a dressing alone.

Modern appliances

These incorporate hypo-allergenic skin protective barriers with soft odour-proof plastic bags in a wide variety of styles. Despite the undoubted advances in appliances made over the years, half of all colostomates have peristomal skin problems and 20 per cent complain of leakage.

Contact dermatitis

This results from allergy to an appliance or adhesive. Effluent dermatitis is more common with ileostomies because of the higher digestive content of the output. Where skin damage is pronounced topical corticosteroids are useful and may be used in combination with a topical antibiotic or antifungal agent where secondary infection has occurred.

Psychological and social problems

The formation of a stoma and loss of the anus is a major violation, causing feelings of shame, degradation, and fear of rejection. The acquisition of anal control in early childhood is important and emotionally charged; its loss as the result of surgery can affect the psyche. The surgeon may be seen as mutilator and the general practitioner preferred as a source of advice for this reason. Ostomates, particularly the elderly, develop a new life-style characterized by conscious control over the range and type of social activity. Patients restrict their range of interests and withdraw from emotional involvement. Fear of odour or leakage leads to social isolation and fears of rejection in up to 75 per cent of ostomates, whilst clinical evidence of depression is present in 30 per cent.

Employment

Although 90 per cent of ileostomates return to work after surgery, the effect of colostomy on subsequent employment is less easy to define because of the effects of age, impending retirement, and underlying disease. Estimates range from 10 to 80 per cent for those able to resume work after colostomy.

A great many misconceptions surround the fitness for ostomates for employment. In fact there are very few restrictions that need to be imposed and the sickness absence records of ileostomates are no different from those of their fellows.

Adequate toilet and washing facilities in the workplace are desirable, and very hot working environments may cause problems with dehydration. Lifting heavy objects in close proximity to the abdominal wall may displace the appliance or damage the stoma. Provided normal personal hygiene and safe work practice are observed there is neither an increased risk of spread of infection from the ostomate nor an increased risk to him or her from agents in the work environment.

Providers of care

The hospital

Before discharge from hospital the patient should have selected a suitable appliance with the help of the nursing staff. He or she should have been taught how to use that appliance and how to care for the stoma to the point of self-reliance. He or she should have been given adequate supplies of appliances on discharge with advice on how to get more. In practice more than 90 per cent receive this level of care. Subsequent out-patient follow up is, however, usually less adequate and one third of patients are dissatisfied with the care they receive. They complain of lack of time, different doctors at each visit, and little contact with the surgeon who did the original operation.

Stoma care nurses

More than 200 stoma care nurses are in post in the UK, with short courses in stoma care provided for community nurses and health visitors. Stoma care nurses are usually based in District General Hospitals and provide a source of help and advice to patients and other health care professionals. Although there are variations in the way these specialist nurses function, they are primarily reactive, responding to demand rather than anticipating need or actively seeking unsolicited problems.

Primary care team

Fewer than 50 per cent of practices organize regular follow-up, either by the general practitioner or the practice nurse, for their stoma patients. The majority of general practitioners are happy to deal with stoma problems, such as diet or psychological disturbance, though many lack confidence in dealing with appliance difficulties. The general practitioner is the preferred source of advice for 'ostomy trouble' for nearly half of all ostomates.

Appliance manufacturers

The representatives of appliance manufacturers have a surprisingly significant involvement in stoma care. This is especially noticeable in areas poorly served by specialist nursing services, such as rural communities. They will examine the stoma and give advice on stoma management as well as organizing the delivery of appliance supplies.

Self-help groups

The best known self-help groups are the Ileostomy Association and the British Colostomy Association. In addition to their customary role of providing advice and promoting research, they also provide 'visitors' to counsel patients before stoma surgery. This activity is of unproven value, though one study suggested that most of those visited felt better as a result. While the Ileostomy Association organizes meetings of its members, the British Colostomy Association is notable for not doing so, since many of its members' primary disease is rectal cancer and their life expectancy is therefore reduced.

The impact of these groups on both ostomates and health professionals has been limited and more needs to be done by these organizations to capture the attention of both consumers and providers of stoma care.

USEFUL ADDRESSES

National Association for Colitis and Crohn's Disease, 98A, London Road, St Albans, Hertfordshire, AL1 1NX, UK. Telephone (0727) 44296.
British Colostomy Association, 15 Station Road, Reading, RG1 1LG, UK. Telephone (0734) 391537.
Ileostomy Association of Great Britain and Ireland, Amblehurst House, Chobham, Woking, Surrey, UK. Telephone (0632) 28099.
Crohn's Disease in Childhood Research Association, 56A, Uxbridge Road, Shepherds Bush, London, W12 8LP, UK. Telephone (081) 949 6209.
The British Digestive Foundation, 3 St Andrew's Place, London NW1 4LB, UK. Telephone (071) 4860341.
National Advisory Service for Parents of Children with a Stoma, 32 Suters Drive, Thorpe Marriott, Taverham, Norwich, Norfolk, UK. Telephone (0603) 860 373.

Several stoma appliance manufacturers produce patient advice leaflets on stoma care and living with a stoma.

FURTHER READING

Bardhan, K. D., Cust, G., Hinchcliffe, R. F. C., Williamson, F. M., Lyon, C., and Bose, K. (1989). Changing patterns of admissions and operations for duodenal ulcer. *British Journal of Surgery*, **76**, 230–6.
Bates, T., Ebbs, S. R., Harrison, M. and A'Hern, R. P. (1991). Influence of cholecystectomy on symptoms. *British Journal of Surgery*, **78**, 964–7.
Gibney, E. J. (1990). Asymptomatic gallstones. *British Journal of Surgery*, **77**, 368–72.
Johnston, G. W., Spencer, E. F. A., Wilkinson, A. T. and Kennedy, T. L. (1991). Proximal gastric vagotomy: follow-up at 10–20 years. *British Journal of Surgery*, **78**, 20–23.
Mayberry, M. K., Probert, C., Sprivastava, E., Rhodes, J., Mayberry, J. F. *et al.* (1992). Perceived discrimination in education and employment by people with Crohn's disease: case control study of educational achievement and employment. *Gut*, **33**, 312–314.
Murray, A., Mitchell, D. C. and Wood, R. F. M. (1992). Lasers in surgery. *British Journal of Surgery*, **79**, 21–6.
Rubin, G. P. (1986). Aspects of stoma care in general practice. *Journal of the Royal College of General Practitioners*, **36**, 369–70.
Rubin, G. P. and Devlin H. B. (1987). The quality of life with a stoma. *British Journal of Hospital Medicine*, **38**, 300–6.
Salky, B. A., Bauer, J. J., Kreel, I., Gelerni, I. M., Gorfine, S. R. (1991). Laparoscopic cholecystectomy: an initial report. *Gastrointestinal Endoscopy*, **37**, 1–4.
Taylor, T. V. (1989). Current indications for elective peptic ulcer surgery. *British Journal of Surgery*, **76**, 427–8.
Wyke, R. J., Aw, T. C., Allan, R. N. and Harrington, J. M. (1939). Employment prospects for patients with intestinal stomas: the attitude of occupational physicians. *Journal of the Society of Occupational Medicine*, **39**, 19–24.

14 The future

Duncan Colin-Jones and Roger Jones

This short chapter highlights topics in gastroenterology which are currently of research and clinical interest, and attempts to predict how they will develop and the impact they may have on management in general practice and at the interface with hospital care. These developments will undoubtedly be driven by many factors, including scientific advance, commercial pressure, social and political changes, and, possibly, changes in the patterns of gastrointestinal disorders. We have already seen how the natural history of important conditions, such as peptic ulceration, has varied over time, how its epidemiology has been changed by widespread prescription of NSAIDs and how the use of potent ulcer-healing agents has transformed the need for surgical intervention. Gastro-oesophageal reflux disease (GORD) has, for reasons that are quite unknown, become a much more significant cause of morbidity in recent years, there is evidence of continuing changes in the pattern and prevalence of Crohn's disease, new challenges for gastroenterologists have been provided by the spread of AIDS and, as the world becomes a smaller place, we are more likely to see conditions which we have traditionally regarded as rare in Western society.

Patients are likely to play an increasingly important role in shaping the development of health care. The Patients' Charter has made explicit the rights of patients in the UK to services and information, the Data Protection Act has given patients access to their medical records and it is likely that demand for negotiated care and, possibly, for better access to investigations and tests will gradually result from these changes. This will, in term, mean that investigations will have to become better-tolerated and will be scrutinized for their accuracy, utility, and cost-effectiveness. One example of this may be the use of flexible sigmoidoscopy, not simply as an investigative procedure, but also as screening method for health checks. Others may include more user-friendly tests for faecal occult blood and non-invasive investigation of upper gastrointestinal problems, such as breath and serological tests for *Helicobacter*.

Linked to the trend towards a more patient-centred health service is a need for patient education about common symptoms. We have seen in earlier chapters how problems such as dyspepsia, reflux symptoms, irritable bowel syndrome, and rectal bleeding are all common in the general population. Although there are unresolved questions about the selection of patients for investigation, the fact that many patients with potentially serious and treatable disorders are experiencing symptoms but not seeking medical advice has clear educational implications. Although, given the remuneration arrangements for general practitioners, it would not be appropriate to encourage consultations for trivial symptoms, there is clearly a need, for example, for a sensitive educational campaign aimed at raising public awareness of the potential significance of symptoms, such as rectal bleeding.

Cost-effective management is going to be the way of the future. This will represent an extension of current pressures from Family Health Service Authorities (FHSAs), through Independent Medical Advisers and also from fund-holding general practices. There are many unanswered questions about what represents cost-effective management. We have already discussed the potential paradoxes in prescribing, in which downward pressure on prescribing costs are not necessarily consistent with rising standards of care. Much more research based on the outcomes of health care is required before we can be confident about what we mean by 'cost-effective', and this is clearly a priority not only for those involved in clinical medicine but also those engaged in health services research and in the purchase and provision of health care in the internal market.

There is likely to be a continued trend towards more routine management of patients with gastrointestinal disorders in general practice and greater selection for those who require referral to a specialized gastroenterology unit. The role of protocols in agreeing selection and treatment criteria between general practitioners and specialists is discussed later, but one possible consequence of this trend is that large practices will set up their own investigative services which may well include flexible sigmoidoscopy, ultrasound scanning (which may also have obstetric and possibly orthopaedic applications) and even upper gastrointestinal endoscopy. General practitioners already play a significant role in providing endoscopic expertise in the hospital setting, with more than 150 general practitioners having clinical assistant or hospital practitioner posts in district general hospitals. A small number of general practitioners have already established upper gastrointestinal endoscopy services based in community hospitals, and a few offer flexible sigmoidoscopy to their patients. These developments are consistent not only with the provision of increasingly comprehensive medical care in general practice, but also with the pressures generated by the internal market, particularly for fund-holding practices working some distance from the nearest district general hospital.

GASTROENTEROLOGY IN GENERAL PRACTICE

Prevention

The use of computers in general practice will, before long, become not merely commonplace but routine. This will provide opportunities to develop and extend patients' databases to include not only information about personal medical history but also about family history and, therefore, risk factors for disease, especially in so-called cancer families, which can be highlighted automatically. This is particularly important in patients with a family history of colorectal cancer. A number of hereditary conditions are associated with an increased individual risk of cancer, including familial adenomatous polyposis, site specific colon cancer and the cancer family syndrome, in which an increased individual risk of colorectal cancer is found in patients whose relatives have had a number of other malignancies, including adenocarcinoma of the uterus, breast, and ovary. These patients and others at high risk, such as those with long-standing inflammatory bowel disease and with a personal history of colorectal neoplasia, can be entered into appropriate screening and surveillance programmes.

Screening

Screening will almost certainly become much more sophisticated. New molecular biological techniques are likely to be applied to select patients who need to enter a regular surveillance programme. This is likely to be true, once again, for colon cancer, where up to five different genetic defects, usually chromosomal deletions, have been found and appear necessary for colon cancer to develop. At first it is likely that colon cancer screening will be offered to patients in the high-risk groups described above but will become more wide-spread, using sophisticated occult blood testing. At present guaiac tests are not particularly well accepted by patients, and more patient-friendly tests for occult gastrointestinal blood loss need to be developed. Genetic probes may be used in the future to make this selection process more specific and more accurate, and could reduce the need for a substantial number of unnecessary negative colonoscopies. Irrespective of the methodologies used, general practice is likely to be the setting for screening high risk groups or for population screening. Current evidence suggests that the uptake of faecal occult blood testing is best when offered by general practitioners during routine consultations for other problems, and the inclusion of faecal occult blood testing in routine health checks has been associated with a lower rate of uptake. This may reflect a number of factors, including the need for better patient awareness of the significance of the test and of the early detection of colorectal neoplasia, but research is clearly needed to define the most cost-effective way of providing good population coverage of this and other screening methods. The introduction of true population screening for colorectal cancer has, at present, been deferred until the results of definitive, large-scale randomized controlled trials are available to determine its utility.

Protocols

It seems likely that increasingly structured care of some gastrointestinal disorders will develop. This may, on the one hand, imply the use of questionnaires for patients to complete, possibly with the development of a scoring system, which may indicate either the need for further investigation or may point towards the possibility of organic disease and the need for symptomatic treatment. Manual scoring systems having been available for some time, and currently patients' age is still regarded as the most important discriminator between a trial of treatment and investigation, with the cut-off at about 45 years. Although in future this is more likely to be done with structured questionnaires and protocols, interest has centred for many years on the use of microcomputer databases as a way of generating lists of diagnostic possibilities and of determining the need for investigation. In general these computer programs have not proved sufficiently compact or robust for use in general practice, and it is more likely that any scoring system will be based on discussion between general practitioners and specialists about patients who, by consensus, are regarded as being in need of investigation.

Audit

It seems likely that FHSAs will be undertaking regular reviews of referral patterns, as well as their current reviews of prescribing costs. This has implications for collaborative, educational, and audit activities taking place between general practices and the local gastroenterology units. Current pressures on these hospital units, related to an ever increasing demand for endoscopy, make it unlikely that, without substantial further funding, there will be time for the close relationships between specialists and general practitioners required for this. Nonetheless, audit is a requirement of both hospital and general practice clinical work now, and audit at the interface between the two is a key area, with major resource implications.

GASTROENTEROLOGY IN THE HOSPITAL

Surgery

The most dramatic change likely to take place in the next few years is almost certainly going to be the microinvasive or minimally invasive technique of laparoscopic surgery. Currently, cholecystectomy is the procedure favoured for this remarkable technique, when four very small incisions are made, a laparoscope is passed, and it is possible to remove the gall-bladder through 1 cm incisions. The result is that the patient spends only a day or two in hospital and returns to work very quickly. It is likely to increase the workload for general practitioners by a small amount, since the convalescent period is short. The patient is usually able to undertake normal activities within two weeks. It certainly should be a very cost-effective form of therapy, because it avoids expensive hospital stays. The technique is likely to be extended to other organs; the appendix has already been tried, resection of the parts of the intestine for benign disease also seems a possibility, and repair of hiatus hernia, highly selective vagotomy, and gastroenterostomy may also be possible through this surgical technique. There are clear implications for training, and also for evaluation; techniques of this kind are not subject to the stringent evaluative requirements of new drugs, despite the fact that they may have just as significant an impact on health and resources. General practitioners need to be aware of these developments because patients will certainly learn about them and will often demand treatments which minimize time lost from work. The availability in different hospitals of different techniques of this kind may well be an important factor in contracting for health care.

Cancer

Planning surgery for patients with cancer is likely to become much more sophisticated. Each patient will have more careful and accurate imaging investigations to detect early, local, and more distant spread. Computerized tomography is increasingly being used for this purpose, but the future may well be with magnetic resonance imaging (MRI) which will help surgeons to see whether a tumour is resectable, how many glands are enlarged and therefore likely to be involved, and whether a limited resection and clearance of glands is required as opposed to radical surgery. These techniques will make surgery much more personalized.

Tumour markers have been found for cancers of the pancreas and colon and these are likely to become more sophisticated. At present they are particularly good at following patients, for example, who have had colon cancer, and looking for evidence of recurrence. At the present time the technology is not good enough to isolate raised levels of the markers to detect cancer at a very early stage, but this may well change with improvements in molecular biological techniques.

Endoscopy

Upper gastrointestinal endoscopy is more accurate than a barium meal and has now become the first choice investigation for upper abdominal symptoms, particularly dyspepsia. Unnecessary duplication will, it is hoped, become a thing of the past, not least because of financial pressures. That will leave endoscopy being undertaken more frequently and radiology probably somewhat less so. This may cause problems in radiology departments in terms of training, as the number of people being referred for gastrointestinal contrast radiology falls. The main problems with endoscopy in the past were its lack of a permanent record, compared with radiographs of barium meals, and the apparent need for sedation for the procedure. This has changed. In many countries there has always been a willingness by the patient to have the procedure undertaken without sedation. This is now being appreciated by the general public in the UK, and more patients are requesting that the procedure should be undertaken with only local pharyngeal anaesthesia. This is proving helpful to gastrointestinal units, which do not have to provide such extensive recovery services, and is helpful to the patient who can carry on with his or her normal activities following the procedure—they will also be able to remember the results from the discussion after the procedure. The other problem, of lack of a permanent record, has now changed because of the introduction and increasingly widespread use of videoendoscopy, where the use of hard computer disks allows the whole record of the examination to be stored. Prints may be taken for documentation in the patient's records and may perhaps form part of the report of the referring doctor. The specialist may also be able to dictate the report during the procedure using a voice-activated recording and reporting system. In the not too distant future such a report may automatically be transmitted to the general practitioner's computer system, providing almost instant communication.

Lasers were heralded as being a very major breakthrough but on the whole they have proved somewhat disappointing. For example, although lasers have been shown to be very effective in reducing gastrointestinal haemorrhage from a bleeding vessel in the base of an ulcer, more recently other techniques such as local injection of substances such as adrenaline and sclerosants, and the use of heater probes, which are very much cheaper, have been shown to be similarly effective. Palliation of stenosing carcinomas of the gastrointestinal tract is another area where the laser has proved useful but by no means perfect, as repeated treatments are often required, in very sick people. Bicap heater probes and stenting with various prostheses offer good alternatives, and laser therapy has not been taken up widely. One particularly exciting area is the place of the photosensitization of tumour cells. An intravenous photosensitizing compound is given and a particular wavelength of laser light is beamed onto the tumour, the cells of which are then damaged because of photosensitization. Superficial lesions may well be cured by this method, but its primary use is for palliation, and in this area it looks very promising.

Biliary problems

It was hoped that the role of the lithotripter, originally introduced as a way of breaking up renal stones with carefully-applied shockwaves, would expand to embrace the treatment of stones in the biliary system. However, until better technology for focusing the energy beam on a gallstone becomes available, the lithotripter is unlikely to have a major impact on gallstone treatment and laparoscopic cholecystectomy has really taken the pressure off the need for such instrumentation. Stones in the bile duct are, however, more difficult for the surgeon doing a laparoscopic cholecystectomy, and endoscopic retrograde cholangiopancreatography (ERCP) is likely to be used in increasing numbers of patients because of the relative inaccessibility of the common bile duct to the surgeon. Newer methods of fragmenting stones within the common bile duct, such as the use of laser sparks, may well make the endoscopist's task, always a difficult one, somewhat easier.

Helicobacter

Over the next few years the role of *Helicobacter pylori* is likely to be better understood. Patients who are infected with this organism can already be detected by urea breath tests or the presence of antibodies in the blood, so it is now possible for the general practitioner to screen for *Helicobacter*. At present we do not know what to do with a positive result but, if prospective studies help us in this respect, we should be able to identify patients who need treatment or further investigation by endoscopy.

Treatment of *Helicobacter* is likely to improve significantly in the next few years. The combination antibiotic regimes have not been widely accepted because they are cumbersome, poorly-tolerated and not particularly efficacious, as problems with drug resistance begin to emerge. There is great interest in the possibility of producing a single drug or a combination compound which is capable of both acid suppression and *Helicobacter* eradication.

There is also intense debate about the possible role of this organism in the development of gastric cancer. If *Helicobacter* is found to have a role in carcinogenesis and if an effective eradication programme can be developed, then there is enormous potential not only for treating ulcers and preventing their recurrence, but also in preventing gastric cancer itself, although this is at present highly speculative.

Inflammatory bowel disease

There is considerable interest in the role of changed bacterial flora in the gastrointestinal tract and, particularly in relation to Crohn's disease, in vascular and haematological factors affecting the intestine. There is, for example, considerable evidence of a hypercoagulable state in inflammatory bowel disease. Whether this is a response to the liberation of inflammatory mediators as part of the disease process or whether it is truly a causative factor in producing intestinal damage remains controversial. However, there is some expectation that both lines of research will lead to the development of more effective and useful drug treatment, which it is hoped will lead to improvement of the quality of life of the patients with inflammatory bowel disease and reduce their need for surgery.

Drug therapy

The pharmaceutical industry is very active in the gastrointestinal field as there are huge rewards for real advances in a system where symptoms are common. It is now possible to control gastric secretion to a remarkable extent with the use of histamine receptor antagonists and proton pump inhibitors. Whilst further additions to these two groups of compounds are quite likely, it is probable that they will have little further impact in this area. Of much greater interest are drugs that modify motility and those to be used in inflammtory bowel disease.

Drugs that modify opioid receptors in the gastrointestinal tract have already been developed and are currently undergoing clinical trial. Additional prokinetic drugs are being actively sought, as it is generally perceived that motility disorders are a common cause of symptoms. If these motility modifying drugs, most of which have actions at 5-hydroxy tryptamine receptors, do prove efficacious they will greatly improve our management of gastrointestinal diseases.

Inflammatory bowel disease is an area in which there is a great deal of research activity, and if the putative organism(s) that lead to the development of Crohn's disease or ulcerative colitis can be found then it follows that drug therapy can be specifically sought. This is a very exciting prospect. Oxygen-free radicals—often produced by the body's own polymorphs—are currently very fashionable. They seem to contribute to a great deal of disease because they are highly reactive and can damage tissues. Drugs are already available for use in the laboratory which modify the development of oxygen-free radicals, and it is likely that similar compounds for use in human subjects will not be long away, and this may well be very valuable for conditions such as pancreatitis.

Functional disorders

Functional disorders, in many ways, represent the largest problem for general practitioners and the area of greatest potential change, although this change may not occur in the direction that most of us would like to see.

It seems possible, for example, that more and more patients with abdominal disorders will seek explanation for their symptoms, particularly as the stresses of life continue to grow and act as triggers to health care seeking and consultation behaviour. There may well, for these reasons, be increased pressures on general practitioners and gastrointestinal services as patients demand accurate diagnoses for their functional gut symptoms.

At present, these are rather difficult to provide, since our concepts and explanations for non-organic abdominal pain are also subject to change and fashion. It is, however, possible that subgroups of patients with functional disorders will emerge, for example certain irritable bowel patients may be found to have a colon colonized with a specific organism, which may have implications for more specific treatment. The interesting possibility that irritable bowel syndrome represents one aspect of a generalized disorder of smooth muscle has been a tantalizing one, both in terms of an explanatory model and a therapeutic opportunity; research interest in this topic is likely to continue.

The stresses of life are unlikely to diminish in the future, and the active support of psychologists both for general practitioners and gastro-enterologists working with patients with functional bowel disorders may well assume greater importance in the years ahead. It is hoped that we can couple this with advances in modern technology and apply both effectively and kindly.

Index